What's in This Book . . .

Chelation (pronounced key-lay-shun) therapy uses chelating agents to literally clean out the arteries; these agents can be administered either orally or intravenously. Chelation therapy is a safe, effective non-surgical treatment that has successfully been used to prevent and treat hardening of the arteries for over forty years in the United States. New evidence indicates that it may also help to control and, in some cases, reverse the effects of arthritis, cancer, stroke, osteoporosis, glaucoma, metal toxicity, irregular heartbeat, senility, gangrene as well as a host of other degenerative illnesses. While the number is growing, there are only a handful of physicians who have taken advantage of its enormous potential.

In this important new book, Dr. Morton Walker explains how chelation works, documents the evidence of its effects, and discusses its oral and intravenous use. Since intravenous treatment is not always necessary, Dr. Walker tells the reader how to use over-the-counter oral chelating nutrients at home. He explains what they are, where to find them, and what dosage to take.

With the publication of this book, the public can now learn about the benefits of this alternative-to-surgery treatment. By implementing some of the information in this book, the reader can improve the quality of life for himself or his loved ones.

THE CHELATION WAY

The Complete Book of Chelation Therapy

Dr. Morton Walker

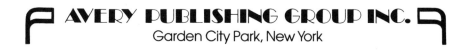
AVERY PUBLISHING GROUP INC.
Garden City Park, New York

The medical information and procedures contained in this book are not intended as a substitute for consulting your physician. All matters regarding your physical health should be supervised by a medical professional.

Cover design: Martin Hochberg and Rudy Shur
Cover photo: Murray Alcosser
In-house editor: Cynthia J. Eriksen
Typesetting: Multifacit Graphics, Keyport, NJ

Library of Congress Cataloging-in-Publication Data

Walker, Morton.
    The chelation way : the complete book of chelation therapy /
Morton Walker.
        p.   cm.
    Includes index.
    ISBN 0-89529-415-X
    1. Atherosclerosis--Chemotherapy. 2. Chelation therapy.
I. Title.
RC692.W2632   1990
616.1'36061--dc20   89-17511
                                                                         CIP

Printed in the United States of America

10 9 8 7 6 5

Contents

Therapy • Assessing the Safety of Chelation
Therapy • Assessing the Efficacy of Medical
Technologies • In the Best Interest of Jackee
Davidson

PART TWO: ORAL CHELATING AGENTS FOR
CARDIOVASCULAR SELF-HELP AT HOME

Dedication

To Audrey Goldman, Executive Director of the Association for Cardiovascular Therapies Inc. (ACT), a humanitarian who gives of her total self for the causes of holistic health, orthomolecular medicine, and chelation therapy without any thought of personal reward. Audrey's satisfaction comes with learning about the successes of those who have gained health from using information provided by her ACT organization.

Foreword

Of all those whose works I read continually, Morton Walker, D.P.M., is the medical journalist whom I hold in the highest esteem. I consider it a privilege to know him as a friend. Dr. Walker's enlightened research, his insightful interpretations, and his straightforward style of writing make each of his books a genuine learning experience for physicians and lay persons alike.

In *The Chelation Way: The Complete Book of Chelation Therapy*, Dr. Walker repeatedly presents the most complicated physiological interactions in an interesting and fascinating manner. I found myself riveted to the manuscript during the entire first reading. Even as co-director of a large medical center for the practice of preventive medicine, I have integrated numerous practical concepts into my clinic's procedures as a result of this book. I always benefit from reading any of the works Dr. Walker has written or from listening to him, either in his lectures or during informal conversations.

Each section of *The Chelation Way: The Complete Book of Chelation Therapy* will fill you with both impact and meaning. Like me, you will no doubt find yourself repeatedly pausing for reflection as you absorb and then apply its information for heightening your own health as well as that of your loved ones. My only regret is that I did not discover Dr. Walker or chelation therapy for cardiovascular disease until after my beloved father, Ronald C. Thedford of Oklahoma City, Oklahoma, suffered his debilitating heart attack fifteen years ago.

I never would have guessed that the ringing of a telephone would have changed my path through life. Early that spring morning I received a call from an employee of my father's telling me that he had been taken to a local hospital emergency room. I heard those dreaded words, "suspected heart attack." Begging for something, anything to be done to save his life, the family was told that he would require further testing. Little did we realize the degree of pain and risk that were involved with those tests. Uninformed, we gave permission for him to have an angiogram. And the inevitable verdict that accompanies angiography held true for my dad, too, after his extensive examinations: "Your options are either to have open heart surgery or to face death."

Any medical treatment is a highly personal issue, especially when life or death is at stake. Weighing the options, and considering the magnitude of his health problem, dad decided to go home, where he thought he might more clearly come to a decision.

Our family panicked! "No surgery," we cried. But his doctors had said that he *must* go through with it. So we wondered and waited and watched as dad, who had been an energetic and active person usually working fourteen to sixteen hours a day, shrunk into a mere ghost of his former self. He could hardly walk across the room without needing to rest. He now slept the number of hours he used to work. He couldn't remember happenings and he didn't remember some lifelong chums. We, his family, watched as this man whom we loved was dying!

One day, a visiting friend left a magazine article for my dad to read. It was about some new therapy called "chelation." After placing several cross-country phone calls, our family located a chelation clinic near to us. Dad went to the chelating physician for consultation. After researching the literature about this treatment, a non-traditional method for the removal of plaque from arteries (the cause of most heart attacks), my father became convinced that chelation was *the* treatment for which he had been searching.

We were not quite so convinced. Family members asked, "Haven't your doctors, the best in our city, told you that it's surgery or death? How can there be a treatment so new that these leading practitioners have no knowledge of it?"

But my dad remained firm in his resolve to take chelation therapy. And loving him very much, we humored the man with, "Whatever makes you happy, makes us happy," all the while fearing that each day was his last.

The chelation treatment program, we learned, consisted of an intravenous fluid with added substances being given over a three- to four-hour period and included dietary changes, vitamin and mineral supplements, and regular daily exercises. It was a simple enough program to follow.

Every day we watched for signs of my dad's change—good or bad. And slowly they occurred. His former ruddy color returned, a healthy glow set in, his step quickened, and his spirits lifted. And our spirits improved, because we saw that his whole quality of life was getting better. We were witnessing our dad's return to us. He is alive and active today.

After experiencing the ordeal that my father and family had endured during this time of crisis, I became interested and quite involved in spreading the word about this chelation treatment. One agonizing part of my father's hospital stay had been when our family asked his physicians, "What can be done to save him?" Their answer, "You have no real choice; it's surgery or eventual death," is a shocking verdict to receive. Especially when I know now that their answer was untrue.

Do you realize how difficult it is to watch someone you love come to a life or death decision? Can you conceive of making such a decision without knowing all the alternatives? Well, people like me aren't letting such awful situations happen anymore. In existence nationwide are groups of lay people, comprised of former and current chelation therapy patients, their appreciative families, and other caring persons in allied health care fields. These grass roots groups of literally thousands of compassionate individuals, who are described in Chapter Seven, give freely of their time, energy, money, and devotion so that others may know of the treatment choices available to victims of cardiovascular and other degenerative diseases. I am the former chairperson of just such a national movement. The primary goal of this organization is to help educate patients, their physicians, and those who wish to stay healthy with preventive measures. The group also furnishes information on alternative options regarding health care. Chelation therapy is definitely a major alternative method.

While no treatment is a panacea, some are better than others. My demand is to at least let the people know what they are. By requiring the most advanced procedures available, we, the medical consuming public, can force our medical community to reevaluate their techniques and upgrade them. Each of us has the right to choose different medical alternatives. We can either accept what the physician says, get additional opinions, or take the option to do absolutely nothing.

Because I know that this treatment has saved my father's life, there will never be enough days or ways for me to tell about the miracle healing power of chelation therapy. I am extremely grateful that chelation therapy is available in our country. Also, I tremendously admire the heroic doctors who provide the treatment for their patients and those who are informing you and me of its existence, why and how it works, who administers it, and all the other education we need to make enlightened judgments.

This is my relationship to chelation therapy. It is a story from the daughter who agonized over the potential loss of her father and saw his life extended by this little known treatment, the woman who has taken chelation therapy herself and experienced marked physical improvement, the wife of a chelating physician who shares gladness and joy with him in the recovery of exceedingly sick patients, the administrator of an expanding medical facility who helps to institute health-sustaining policy, the health educator who realizes the need to send forth the message of available preventive medical care, and the mother who wants most of all the healthiest of worlds for her children and for future generations.

If the principles of health care as exemplified in *The Chelation Way: The Complete Book of Chelation Therapy* would be accepted by our culture, I believe the quality and duration of life could be immeasurably enhanced. However, without acting on these printed words, all the information in the world would be of little value. Now the word is out. The option of chelation therapy is ready for use. The choice is yours.

When you have finished reading this book or using it for reference, share it with a loved one or friend. The life you save will certainly be theirs.

Skoshi Thedford Farr
Genesis Medical Center
Oklahoma City, Oklahoma

Preface

Chelation therapy performs its healing by reversing hardening of the arteries. As yet the treatment is not generally accepted by the health care establishment for the clearing of clogged blood vessels. Instead, organized medicine tries to limit the treatment's use to lead poisoning, snake bite, and other types of toxicity reactions. For this reason few victims of degenerative diseases having blocked blood flow as their underlying pathology know that a valid alternative to standard but sometimes ineffective medical procedures exists. Consequently, people wise in the ways of alternative health care have cried out for a book such as *The Chelation Way: The Complete Book of Chelation Therapy* to be written, read, and passed from person to person. Information furnished here tends to save individuals' lives, limbs, and much unhappiness.

Chelation therapy was introduced into the United States in 1948 after its development in Germany in the early 1930s. The treatment is well recognized by medical authorities around the world as the definitive recourse against heavy metal toxicity, radiation toxicity, digitalis intoxication, snake venom poisoning, and heart arrhythmias. Even with our medical establishment's non-recognition for its best effect, the treatment's most important application is for preventing or reversing heart and artery pathology derived from diminished blood circulation.

Specifically designated for correcting circulatory difficulties, chelation therapy has already been administered to over 500,000 Americans and about one million Canadians, Russians, Europeans, Australians, South Americans, and other people around the world who had been suffering from hardening of the arteries. It has been given to more than double those numbers for the elimination of heavy metal toxicity. The treatment is safe, relative to other modalities that are as commonly used.

I receive letters and telephone calls from some of those patients who have been restored to health as a result of reading my writings on chelation therapy. In other cases, people worried about the cardiovascular problems of friends, relatives, or themselves request information from me that goes beyond what they have learned from my books, magazine articles, and lectures. Or, they may want to speak to me to get a physician referral, dosage form, opinion, or some other item. In all cases, I try to inform people that I do not sell treatment, prescribe drugs or nutrients, or practice medicine. I am strictly a medical journalist who tries to provide information that is not usually available in the lay press.

I have been averaging five phone calls or letters daily since 1978 when in Connecticut, I became one of three people who incorporated the Association for Cardiovascular Therapies Inc. (ACT). I was the first president of ACT. The writer of this book's foreword, Skoshi Farr, was ACT's second president. This non-profit, charitable organization provides medical consumer support and education on alternative forms of healing. I usually turn over my reader response to ACT for furnishing the appropriate replies. You will find more information about ACT, including its location, in Chapter Seven.

Letters of query that arrive at my desk come mostly from the loved ones of heart attack victims, potential amputees, those facing coronary artery bypass surgery, and others just curious about chelation therapy. They frequently want to know where to get intravenous injections with the synthetic amino acid, EDTA, that reverses arterial pathology. Sometimes they want to know of generic names, brand names, dosages, addresses, and other intelligence about oral chelating agents. I fill in missing information where possible, although I do advise my questioner that almost everything that I know about chelation therapy is written in my books, journal articles, magazine articles, and booklets or delivered in my public lectures.

Yet, the field is ever changing. My attendance at the semi-annual meetings of the American College of Advancement in Medicine Inc. provides me with a continual updating of scientific information. I incorporate the updating in the newest editions of my published works or I may write another book, booklet, pamphlet, or magazine article or I revise my current lecture on chelation therapy. This book reflects such an updating. It is totally new and does not repeat anything that I have written heretofore.

For three decades, for example, traditional physicians who practice mainstream medicine but really prefer to be exponents of chelation therapy have demanded that scientifically conducted clinical trials be utilized to demonstrate the treatment's efficacy. Those clinical trials have finally been performed, and they are presented in Chapters Four and Five. Moreover, nowhere else is there published such a complete report on existing and available oral chelating agents as those detailed in this book's Part Two. Oral chelators consist of nutrients, supplements, foods, drugs, and certain in-between products called "nutras" that act as pharmaceutical nutrients (or nutritional pharmaceuticals).

Some of the described oral chelators are not approved for American import or usage in this country by the United States Food and Drug Administration. Intravenous chelation therapy and its associated orally administered chelating products have been praised for their therapeutic value. Many people have testified to the health benefits they have received from use of such chelation treatment. A number of case histories and direct patient and doctor quotes, in fact, are cited in this book illustrating how the treatments, foods, and pills have been helpful to relieve the symptoms and signs of disease. Yet, we wish to caution against letting our publication become any kind of substitute for proper medical attention. In other words, don't let *The Chelation Way: The Complete Book of Chelation Therapy* become a replacement for competent medical advice. We definitely recommend that you seek such medical attention from a holistic physician who makes chelation therapy a part of his treatment regimen when it is called for. Certainly avoid the narrow-minded physician-politician who condemns out of hand the use of chelation treatment when he or she has never administered it or taken it for his own hardening of the arteries. Then he or she is playing the political game of physician peer review when that doctor-politician doesn't really know what he is talking about. Such a physician-politician should himself be condemned and possibly sued for medical malpractice when he fails to present chelation treatment to the patient as a viable alternative to the other procedures in the medical marketplace.

We also warn you about placing too much emphasis on chelation therapy as the only form of prevention or treatment plan to be engaged in. Watch out that you don't reject mainstream medical methods just because they are traditional techniques.

Nothing written in *The Chelation Way: The Complete Book of Chelation Therapy* should be construed as prescribing therapeutically for any health problem. What I have written here is strictly for informational purposes. My observation is that organized medicine has a stranglehold on the kind of health care information that gets published; therefore, it is necessary for lay persons to receive education about medical aspects other than what is good public relations for the professional health care establishment.

On a personal note, my wife and I have taken chelation therapy ourselves. To date, I have received fifty-eight intravenous feedings averaging 210 minutes each. My wife also has taken many treatments. Both of us intend to receive more injections. We do this not for the correction of any symptomatology, but strictly for life extension. We know that cleaning out our arteries of accumulated plaque material and giving the cells a chance to function more normally will allow us to live nearer to the full complement of mankind's 120 years.

And both of us supplement our diets with copious quantities of oral chelating agents, primarily vitamins, minerals, herbs, fatty acids, enzymes, protomorphogens, fiber, an occasional hormone supplement, amino acids, antioxidants, agents against free radicals, nutras, many food factors, and rarely any drugs except those dedicated to tissue or cellular enhancement in the form of body nutrition or waste disposal. You might consider a similar life extension program for yourself. Of course, it should include the various forms of chelation therapy—intravenous and oral—that I describe in this book.

Morton Walker, D.P.M.
Stamford, Connecticut

PART ONE
The Intravenous Infusion Form of Chelation Therapy

CHAPTER ONE
What If You or Your Loved One Has Clogged Arteries?

Would you be interested in knowing of a safe, effective, tested, legal, non-surgical treatment that helps to remove blockage of human arteries?

Would you want to have this dependable procedure and its nutritional compounds available as a substitute for dangerous medical procedures that are directed against relieving symptoms but not correcting disease?

Would you like to eliminate questionable health-care methods such as life-threatening open heart surgery, the unnecessary amputation of gangrenous limbs, the complication-ridden cleaning of neck arteries, the use of powerful cardiovascular drugs with their myriad side effects, and other serious, painful, and expensive medical methods that do little for the patient but much for the pocketbooks of medical specialists, pharmaceutical companies, and hospitals?

Would you want your family physician to know all about this comfortable correction and set you to following a lifestyle that could add twenty to thirty years more to the time you have to live?

Would you be dubious if an informed person told you that some cardiologists, endocrinologists, internists, and other high-priced practitioners didn't have any knowledge of this trustworthy treatment and might refuse to prescribe it even if they did?

Would you be surprised to learn that the technique's easy application takes little skill, could be administered by a technician, and merely requires a physician's knowledgeable supervision?

Would you be shocked to learn that the ordinary medical doctor in your community who wants to bring this treatment to his or her patients is pressured out of doing so through the threat of colleague criticism, formal peer review, refusal of health insurance companies to pay his patients' claims, loss of university appointments, loss of hospital affiliation, loss of patient referrals from fellow doctors, loss of professional liability (malpractice) insurance, loss of medical association membership, and possible loss of his license to practice medicine?

If you have an emergency need for such a treatment, would you feel frustration and anger at not being informed of its existence when your physician presented the ways and means to overcome your health problem so that you might live a little longer?

SAVED FROM ALZHEIMER'S-LIKE SENILITY

Suppose you and others who love her have concluded that there is no way your elderly mother can remain at home unsupervised. You see that her mind is gone. The doctor thinks that she is suffering from senility, an Alzheimer's-like syndrome, or some other form of senile dementia.

While you remember how a few years ago she had been so mature and level-headed, alert and vivacious, always joking, clear thinking, and physically active, now the woman is forgetful, depressed, argumentative, childish, lethargic, and terribly weak. She has frequent accidents, such as spilling hot cooking oil down her legs. She loses things, like the time her house keys were misplaced and all the locks had to be changed. She usually gets lost, including her disconcerting inability to find the bathroom in her own home. Consequently, she has reverted to infantilism by wetting her bed and at times defecating in her clothes.

You and other family members have come to a decision: your elderly mother must enter a nursing home, where she will probably vegetate until she dies. You are distressed with this decision, but the "experts" have said that there is nothing else to be done, since no known treatment for senility exists.

Then, while arrangements are being made for the woman's entry into the convalescent hospital, you stumble upon a book about some marvelous treatment that acts like a kind of gentle Drano™ to unblock clogged blood vessels in the body and brain. You bring this book to your mother's physician and inquire about the procedure. "Will it work?" you ask. The doctor, an honorable person but in the dark about its action, is likely to feel threatened by medical questions he or she cannot answer. Not uncommonly, a traditionally trained physician practicing in the medical mainstream will come down on what he fails to be up on and so will declare that such a treatment is "nonsense" or will label it "quackery."

This is exactly what happened to Judith Normant of Tulsa, Oklahoma, in 1974, when she was sadly arranging the permanent transfer of her senile parent to a nursing home. The daughter received information on chelation therapy and sought advice of the family doctor, himself elderly, a geriatrician who had tended to Judith's mother, 80-year-old Mrs. Nancy Curtis, for more than forty years. This old-timer, mired in medical orthodoxy, used some colorful language regarding the non-traditional treatment that Mrs. Normant described.

But the daughter pursued the subject and contacted another physician who was listed in the book's appendix along with those colleagues providing chelation therapy. As it happens, this chelating physician, Charles H. Farr, M.D., Ph.D. of Oklahoma City, Oklahoma, was chairman of the American Board of Chelation Therapy, the medical specialty organization that trains, tests, and certifies doctors to give the treatment. On her own, with no financial assistance from Medicare, Judith Normant brought Mrs. Curtis to Dr. Farr for chelation therapy. She loved her mother enough to go that little extra, trying to bring back the old lady to nearly what she had been.

Nancy Curtis received thirty intravenous chelation injections plus quantities of oral chelating agents administered by Dr. Farr. Her period of treatment lasted from June 5, 1974, to July 11, 1974. Judith Normant reports that she witnessed all kinds of improvement in her mother's behavior during that time. The old woman again recognized loved ones and friends. She became aware of her surroundings. Immediately Mrs. Curtis became continent during the day and also stopped voiding in bed, since at night she was able to navigate from her bedroom to the bathroom. Instead of lingering in night clothes, she rose in the morning and got dressed for the day. Her personality turned cheerful, and short-term memory returned so that she began once again to speak of recent events, people she had met, and current holidays to celebrate. She started telling jokes with a quick wit and a ready laugh. Cooking and recipes became her occupation once more; Judith took the woman on auto drives and shopping excursions to the supermarket—the first time in two years that Mrs. Curtis had engaged in this activity.

Everything was going well for the patient by the end of the current series of thirty chelation treatments. (See Figure 1.1.) Dr. Farr decided to end the injections for a few months while Mrs. Curtis continued on her own to take oral chelators in pill form. Then, tragedy struck the old lady. Her stepson by a previous marriage, a man whom she had raised from boyhood, was killed in an automobile accident. He had lived in a distant city, and it was necessary for Nancy Curtis to arrive there quickly to attend his funeral.

Inasmuch as there had been no love or any relationship between the Curtis family and the family of Nancy's first husband, no one in Tulsa felt the need to travel such a distance for the stepson's funeral. But Mrs. Curtis wanted to go, and she did fly across the country—alone! She also returned home without mishap, something quite remarkable for a person who just ten weeks before had almost been given up as the hopeless victim of senile dementia resulting from hardening of the arteries of the brain.

Mrs. Nancy Curtis is still enjoying a productive life today, more than ten years after her comeback from the living death of (Alzheimer's-like) senility. She maintains herself with occasional physician-administered intravenous feedings using the protein ingredients of chelation therapy. She also eats an exceedingly healthy diet of vegetables, fruits, whole grains, and not much animal protein. More than this, every day it is her ritual with meals to swallow handfuls of chelating agents in the form of nutritional supplements and some pharmaceuticals. Her mind is clear so that she knows the exact components and dosages of each pill she takes. Exercise is an essential part of the woman's chelation program, too, and daily she manages to get in three miles of vigorous walking around her neighborhood, not necessarily performed all in one hike. When the

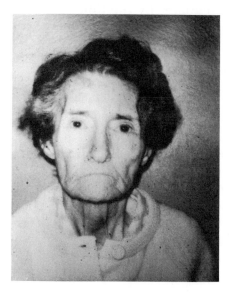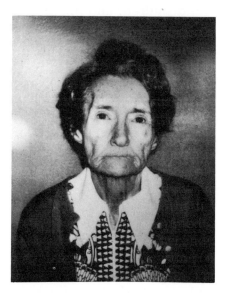

1. Shown is Mrs. Nancy Curtis, an 80-year-old lady suffering from senility and exhibiting symptoms of infantile withdrawal. She has cerebral arteriosclerosis. The picture was taken by her physician, Charles H. Farr, M.D., Ph.D. of Oklahoma City, just prior to his administering intravenous chelation therapy to her on June 5, 1974. At this time, Mrs. Curtis is not cognizant of where she is, who she is, or anything else about herself. Three days before this date she had been lying in bed curled into the fetal position, babbling like a baby, and defecating on herself.

2. Five weeks later, July 11, 1974, after Nancy Curtis received chelation treatment, she improved considerably in mind and body. Notice her eyes! They show the woman to be much more oriented to her surroundings, to who she is, and to what she is doing. In fact, one month after this picture was taken by Dr. Farr, the patient booked passage on an airplane, flew to attend the funeral of her stepson, and returned without mishap, all by herself. This was a remarkable feat for a formerly senile person newly released from hardening of the arteries to her brain.

**Figure 1.1.   Improvement in awareness
due to intravenous chelation therapy.**

weather is stormy, she remains indoors and bounces on her rebounding device, a minitrampoline that she uses faithfully. At 90 years, Mrs. Nancy Curtis, whom Dr. Farr reported on to me during the summer of 1983, is in fine shape. She is enjoying her great-grandchildren, and one of them is pregnant. By the time you read this, Mrs. Curtis will probably be playing with her great-great-grandchild.

LEGS NEED NOT BE AMPUTATED

Suppose that your blood flow is so poor to your lower limbs, the doctor says you have no hope to live unless you have them cut off. It's a devastating idea. For your entire life you have been active and, until the past few years, relatively athletic. Suddenly now, you must face daily living without the ability to get around and do things for yourself. You see yourself pushing your legless body about on a skate board, selling pencils on street corners. "It's better to die," says the small voice within you.

But you can't wait to die, because the leg pain is forcing you toward accepting the amputation operation. Not only are you faced with the psychological trauma of being without lower extremities, but you can't stand the unending pain in your legs. Narcotics and other types of pills seem to do little to kill the pain. What's the problem? Poor circulation is bringing on peripheral nerve irritation that sometimes has you groaning with the constant deep aching and frequent sharp stabs of pain. Your muscles, connective tissues, bones, blood vessels, joints, cartilage, and other structures in the lower limbs are crying out for oxygen. The blood is supposed to carry oxygen from your lungs to the legs, but your oxygenated blood can't get down to the extremities because their arteries are overly narrowed or blocked.

Do you think that my description is far-fetched or too dramatic? Then let me introduce you to Peter B. Donaldson of Mill Valley, California. Mr. Donaldson provided his story of lower limb pain and potential gangrene for publication here, through his chelation therapy physician, Robert Haskell, M.D., of San Francisco. Dr. Haskell is a member of the American College of Advancement in Medicine, and you will find a listing for his office on page 256.

Peter Donaldson wrote me a letter for publication, saying: "Peripheral vascular disease has been a devastating experience for me. Two accepted treatments are bypass surgery and amputation. Another medical treatment which is not commonly known is chelation therapy. This story gives an account of my experience with these various treatment modalities. They were the beginning of a long journey that was to involve various kinds of surgeries, crutches, walkers, canes, and physical pain that I endured in an effort to remain whole."

Throughout his body the man suffered with diminution in the width of the central channels in his arteries, which ordinarily allow blood to flow along the circulatory tree of his cardiovascular system. Such blood vessel narrowing is common among middle-aged American men, because general lifestyle for this patient population is among the unhealthiest on planet Earth. This patient population is committing a slow form of suicide by eating a high-fat diet and too much animal protein in the form of pork and beef, drinking alcoholic beverages to excess, consuming insufficient quantities of complex carbohydrates and an overabundance of sugared and starchy products, smoking tobacco or marijuana, and taking on numerous other risk factors. They usually die prematurely, in the range of one half to two thirds of the number of years they are genetically coded to live (up to 120).

When Peter Donaldson began with the difficulties he is about to describe, he was only 40 years old. His admission is that previous to being struck with disease symptoms, he had indulged in "the revolutionary drug culture." Donaldson smoked approximately four packs of cigarettes a day for over twenty-five years. He drank booze and beer to excess and irregularly ate meals that included a diet high in fatty hamburgers. This type of lousy lifestyle caused his arteries to clog and harden with atherosclerotic plaque, which is the junk material that often lines the inside of blood vessel walls. Atherosclerotic plaque tends to narrow the blood channels and to block blood flow.

"In 1979 I had a femoral-popliteal bypass graft on my left leg, from groin to ankle," Donaldson wrote. A femoral-popliteal bypass graft is a surgical procedure performed to skirt or shunt blocked blood vessels, in this case the femoral artery and the popliteal artery, to relieve an obstruction of circulating blood to other structures in the leg.

"In 1980 I had angioplasty on my right leg and was advised that I should have the same procedure on my face. I declined the facial surgery." Angioplasty is plastic reconstructive surgery performed upon arteries and veins that have been damaged from degenerative disease or by an accident.

"In February 1982 my femoral-popliteal bypass seemingly became clogged overnight, and I was in critical condition." Donaldson was rushed to the hospital as a measure to prevent the limb from sustaining gangrene. The failed bypass graft eliminated the entire blood supply to his left leg.

"The emergency room doctor threatened me with a left below-the-knee amputation but decided instead to first perform a streptokinase drip." Streptokinase is a powerful drug that breaks down blood clots. It is administered by intravenous infusion for arterial blockages, but the danger is that spontaneous hemorrhaging will occur, because the entire clotting mechanism in a patient is degraded. All kinds of complications could take place such as anaphylaxis, fever, and severe uncontrolled internal bleeding.

"I was violently opposed to both procedures (the amputation and the intravenous streptokinase infusion) but found myself powerless in the face of modern medical expertise. While on the streptokinase I began bleeding internally," said Donaldson. My investigation of the patient's hospital history turned up that during the intravenous feeding, his heart had stopped beating, and he was pronounced dead in the emergency room. This indicates that he probably suffered an anaphylactic allergic reaction to the streptokinase. The drip was stopped at once inasmuch as his life had been snuffed out, but heroic measures by the emergency room personnel brought him back to life.

"I received multiple surgical operations and fifty-five pints of blood within a twenty-four-hour period," Donaldson continued. "This rendered me helplessly disabled and in intensive care for about twelve days. Thereafter, I remained in severe pain and unable to walk or work for a living.

"Due to the continued support of friends, family and months of physical rehabilitation, by December 1982 I was mobile enough to use a cane. I was able to walk approximately two level city blocks before severe cramping struck in both of my legs. At this time, the doctors working on my case strongly urged that I undergo a below-the-knee amputation of my left leg. The final blow came," Donaldson said, "when I consulted a top physician in the vascular field. He pronounced that I had only about six months to a year before the left leg would be totally dead (gangrenous). At this time, my foot was white, cold, and my big toe was giving me extreme pain. I had little hope at this point of retaining my body intact.

"Near the end of December 1982, a new glimmer of hope showed on the horizon. Because a doctor once suggested that I had Buerger's disease, a friend picked up a booklet (*Dr. Donsback Tells You What You Always Wanted to Know About Chelation*) on chelation therapy, written by Morton Walker, D.P.M. My friend bought it for me from the local health food store and presented it as a gift during the Christmas holidays. Here, at last, I saw another alternative I could use.

"My efforts to find a chelating physician with whom I could trust my health led me to the office of Dr. Robert Haskell in San Francisco," Donaldson stated. "I found Dr. Haskell to be a caring person with a gentle soul and a twinkle in his eye. He listened to my story just as I'm telling it now. He told me the truth about my condition's potential outcome. Because of my previous surgical history and the current poor status of my lower left leg, the amount of improvement we could expect was questionable. After consulting with members of his staff, it was decided among us that I could always resort to amputation. For the present, we agreed to try to save my leg. Thus, my chelation treatments began the following week.

"I must confess that years of surgeries and sporadic physical incapacitation have left me drained financially. I just have no money. Dr. Haskell believed that if my leg was to be saved, the treatment had to be started immediately. He made no demands for payment on me but merely said, 'It will work out.' I was very touched by his concern," said Donaldson, "and felt that at last someone in this work actually cared. In fact, everything really has worked out financially, since my health insurance company has been paying the medical bills like clockwork.

"I began my chelation therapy on February 4, 1983. As of today, August 19, 1983, I have received forty-eight treatments. During this time, my body has gone through several transformations. By May 1st I was able to walk without my cane. The cramping in my legs does not occur now until after I have walked at least six level city blocks or about three San Francisco uphill blocks. The leg cramps then subside within two minutes, and I can continue on. At times I do feel muscle cramping at rest, but this can be massaged away within about five minutes.

"After the disaster following the streptokinase drip in 1982, I was told by medical authorities that I had renal failure," Donaldson continued. "Naturally, a concern of mine when I started chelation treatment was the potential kidney damage noted in the three other books on chelation therapy written by Dr. Morton Walker [*The Healing Powers of Chelation Therapy, Chelation Therapy,* and *The Chelation Answer*]. Not only have I not noted any kidney problems due to the chelation, but the prechelation pain which was centered around the kidney area has completely subsided.

"My most serious vascular malady, my lower left leg and foot, has improved dramatically. To reiterate, in February 1982 a below-the-knee amputation was strongly recommended. My left foot had sores that would not heal and was without pulses. My chelation therapy began one year later, in February 1983. The sores cleared remarkably well and are completely gone now. Indeed, in June 1983, my former vascular surgeon who had so strongly advised that I have my leg cut off, examined me and felt a pulse on the top of my left foot. In amazement he stated, 'At this point, I would not amputate the leg.' "

Peter B. Donaldson concluded, "Because I was fortunate enough to read some information about chelation therapy, it looks like I have won my fight to remain whole."

In a follow-up communication, Dr. Robert Haskell wrote, "This letter is an addendum to the history of Peter Donaldson. The patient reports on this date that he has been completely asymptomatic. The paresthesias that had run down the back of his legs are not there anymore. For the first time in years, the man has been able to experience an erection. He no longer has pain in his great toe or elsewhere in his body. He is very thrilled . . . and so are we!"

Donaldson is helping himself as well, and isn't depending solely on the chelation treatment to reverse hardening of the arteries in his lower body. He has stopped his excessive drinking of hard liquor and only during social occasions takes a bit of white wine. The man has also stopped smoking cigarettes. And he takes nutritional supplements plus other chelating agents by mouth following each meal.

SELF-RESCUED FROM HAVING OPEN HEART SURGERY

Suppose you are working the evening shift at your occupation and have just finished dinner with a cool glass of lemonade when a sharp heart pain strikes you in the chest. The pain radiates into the throat, up your neck, down your left arm, and burns like a hot poker in the middle of your breast. There is no doubt in your mind from all that you've read and heard from others that your heart is now under attack. And in that moment before collapsing, you realize that those small suffocating periods of pain you had been experiencing for the last few weeks were not recurrences of indigestion after all, but rather angina pectoris.

While I could be describing anyone's heart attack here, this one is all the more significant because it happened to a family physician, 63-year-old Floyd B. Coleman, M.D., of Waterloo, Indiana. May 12, 1981, while serving on emergency room duty at Cameron Memorial Hospital in Angola, Indiana, Dr. Coleman was stricken by severe anginal pain of the preinfarction type. Infarction means that an area of tissue in the man's heart was being deprived of its blood supply because of a clot within the artery ordinarily bringing oxygen and nutrition to the involved area. The attack hit at 6:00 p.m., and Dr. Coleman was assigned to attend emergency room patients until eight o'clock the next morning.

Coleman admits to being a tough old bird. He diagnosed himself, popped some nitroglycerine under his tongue every two hours to relieve the symptoms, and continued working. "My heart problem was of a peculiar type. It's the kind called Prinzmetal's angina and strikes at night. During the current attack, every time I laid down between patients, my heart pain would awaken me out of a doze. I would have to move my legs to take a little load off the heart muscle so as to get relief. Lower extremity movement acted as a sort of heart pump to push up the blood and return it to the heart. A few times during my shift, the night duty nurse called me to attend an emergency. This physical movement, combined with the nitroglycerine, allowed me to get through my hospital shift. If I had been called to a really serious emergency case, I would have asked for help from a relief doctor.

"I came under the care of an excellent cardiologist-internist at Fort Wayne, Indiana, who ordered angiograms taken of me at Fort

Wayne Lutheran Hospital," said Dr. Coleman. "The angiograms revealed that I had 100 percent occlusion of a major coronary artery and 90 to 95 percent occlusions of the rest of my coronary arteries. The cardiologist recommended that I quickly undergo open heart surgery in order to save my life. He wasted no words on pleasantries and warned that I only had a 50 percent chance of living for thirty days more unless I went under the knife for at least a triple coronary artery bypass operation. It was a black prognosis and was presented to me with a hard sell.

"The angiograms had been performed Friday afternoon, and the cardiologist arrived early Saturday morning to give me the bad news," Dr. Coleman continued. "I became anxious and depressed as I lay flat on my back. My operation was scheduled in three days, for the following Tuesday. It was nothing that I wanted because my brother had died within one month of having undergone open heart surgery at the Mayo Clinic. And his wife had died on the table during her open heart surgery, performed at the University Hospital in Louisville, Kentucky. I did not like one bit that my heart would be stopped for six hours while the surgeons took the saphenous vein out of my leg and patched it into my heart arteries.

"But I weighed all the facts in my case. I was in a bad way. Even brushing my teeth had been bringing on angina pain. I had no work tolerance at all. I was a typical type-A behavior person," the physician-patient said. The *type-A personality* wages a continual battle against time and other people. He or she races to perform tasks even when he does not have to—an overly conscientious, constantly busy, obsessively punctual and highly competitive personality. Dr. Coleman is a workaholic—putting himself on call for practicing medicine twenty-four hours a day. He is currently coroner of DeKalb County, Indiana, and formerly served in the state legislature. He has been married to the same woman for forty-three years, has eight children, flies a plane, and cuts wood with a chain saw for recreation. He can't stand not to be busy doing productive enterprises.

"About ten years ago, Richard Willard, M.D., a maverick-type physician with whom I was acquainted, introduced chelation therapy to the staff at Cameron Memorial Hospital. It was incorporated as a part of the emergency room procedures. Inasmuch as I was on duty in the E.R. pretty regularly then, he asked me to be responsible for its administration. By way of coaching, Dr. Willard gave me a book to read on the subject. He had the patients come into the hospital emergency room to get chelated, and every Sunday it fell to me to give them their infusions," Dr. Coleman said. "There was no one on the hospital staff opposed to giving patients the treatment. The health insurance companies paid the medical bills for it— a procedure they labelled "chemical endarterectomy" or chemotherapy for arteriosclerosis. And it seemed all right to me to give this treatment. The patients with heart trouble appeared to thrive on it."

At our August 23, 1983 interview, Dr. Coleman told me that he had prayed a lot about the decision he was being forced to make. "I laid these problems before God and tried to trust Him for guidance and healing." It was then that Dr. Coleman was led to leave the hospital and to cancel his appointed coronary artery bypass operation.

"I felt that I should give myself chelation intravenous treatments and proceeded to take them once daily for four consecutive days and then three per week. With getting only seventeen treatments, I obtained marked relief from my heart pains. The angina went away. I then continued to provide myself with chelation therapy twice a week until I have received fifty intravenous treatments. Next I reduced the number to once a week until I had nearly sixty-five infusions running through my blood vessels. I have been continuing with one treatment every two or three months. By now I have taken seventy-four chelation injections. In this way, I have bypassed the triple bypass, which would have put my life on the line and would have cost me about forty thousand dollars. I continue to take chelation therapy, following a strict diet in accordance with the program set forth by the American College of Advancement in Medicine, including no refined sugars, no caffeine, no nicotine, no red meat, and no fat. I have dropped thirty pounds in excess weight. And I take my nutritional and pharmaceutical chelating agents faithfully," said Dr. Coleman.

He runs a full medical practice six days a week. "About fifty patients pass through my doors daily. I keep my staff of nurses hopping. Even in my younger years, I hadn't felt as well as I do today," said this chelating physician.

CHAPTER TWO
What Is Chelation Therapy?

In 1968, at age 52, Isadore Resnick of West Hartford, Connecticut, an entrepreneur in the amusement business, was the first person in the Hartford metropolitan area to undergo a coronary artery bypass operation. It was, in fact, the first such procedure that cardiac surgeon Henry Low, M.D., had ever performed at Hartford Hospital. Dr. Low referred to his patient as "the bravest man I've ever known." Mr. Resnick described himself to me as "foolhardy." The heart patient declared that he never again would consent to being a guinea pig for a surgeon untested in a procedure as hazardous as open heart surgery.

Currently costing about fifty thousand dollars for hospital care and surgeon's skill, coronary artery bypass surgery tries to solve the blockage of arteries supplying blood to the heart muscle. The blockage is caused by a buildup of material called "plaque" on the inner and middle walls of blood vessels, especially the coronary arteries. The plaque causes them to narrow.

Such blockage forces the heart to work harder. The long-term result can be a heart attack, before and after which many victims experience chest pains known as angina pectoris.

Coronary artery bypass surgery involves using portions of the saphenous vein from a leg to bypass blocked heart arteries. Until now, when chelation therapy has been growing in popularity as a viable substitute, this dangerous heart operation had been considered essential for victims of severe angina. The open heart patching procedure was also applied to similar diseases of the arteries supplying blood to the left ventricle of the heart, which pumps oxygen-rich blood to the body.

Isadore Resnick underwent his coronary bypass because of the acute angina that he had been experiencing for a year before the operation. The pain had become progressively harsher, more frequent, and debilitating. It was coming on with less and less physical effort. He found it difficult even to cross a suburban street. Yet, another physician, whom Resnick no longer considers his family doctor, called the pain a mental problem and prescribed valium.

When the patient could not function normally any longer—was unable to talk on the phone for more than three minutes without feeling heart pain—his physician finally sent him for coronary angiography.

Taking an angiogram of the heart involves using a dye that the angiologist injects into the arteries so as to visualize the coronary arteries on X-ray film. A thin catheter tube is snaked through an artery in the arm or neck to eventually reach the heart. It slides into the aorta, and the dye is specifically placed to fill the tiny coronary arteries that supply the heart muscle.

The angiogram taken of Resnick revealed his total blockage of the right coronary artery. Thus, he acceded to becoming the first Hartford-area bypass patient.

The operation did not work well. The patient experienced the same symptoms as before. The shock of undergoing a life-threatening procedure, however, caused the man to completely change his unhealthy lifestyle. In 1969, the health movement in the United States had not yet reached the popular proportions it has now, and Resnick had to do a lot of investigating among health food exponents to learn how to eat and behave amidst society's high technology living.

"I reduced the fat content of my diet and ate more complex carbohydrates," Resnick told me in our recorded interview. "I took vast quantities of vitamins, minerals, and other nutritional supplements [which, unknown to him at the time, actually were oral chelating agents]. I forced myself to take long, slow walks every day." All this the patient did on his own without any coaching from the surgeon. It was rare at that time to have a physician take an interest in his patient's lifestyle, inasmuch as most physicians are taught how to cope with disease and not how to keep a person well.

The cardiologist that Resnick went to for checkups expressed amazement at his patient's steady improvement over time. This doctor described his other patients as either staying the same following the open heart operation, which was the best they could hope for, or getting worse. But Resnick's electrocardiograms taken through the years 1970 to 1977 repeatedly improved until they looked almost normal.

"The cardiologist told me," reported Resnick, "that the credit for this improvement was not a result of his treatment but belonged to what I was doing for myself. The doctor said, 'I don't know what you're doing, and I'm not interested in knowing.' Obviously, he wanted me to keep doing it."

Life and health were uneventful for the man until the summer of 1978, when he experienced a sudden recurrence of his symptoms of ten years previous. The unexpected onset of stabbing breast pain made breathing difficult for him. Then he found himself unable to walk from one room to the next without taking nitroglycerine under the tongue. He could not converse for more than a minute without feeling searing pain in the chest. He was forced to write on a pad to express his needs.

The man's wife, Helen, told me that she lived in a constant state of anxiety not knowing when her husband might be hit by a massive heart attack. "I laid awake beside him most of the night just to make sure he was breathing," she said. "I would feel the area of his heart or put my hand around his wrist to check if his pulse was beating. If he snored, I was delighted. I became extremely nervous. Women who live with this sort of situation will know exactly what I went through."

A doctor suggested to Resnick that he undergo another coronary angiogram and subsequent bypass operation—something the patient wanted no part of. It was then that Resnick began investigating alternative forms of treatment. He telephoned me, because someone had suggested to him that I may have useful information about a chemical Roto-Rooter™ treatment to replace the open heart surgery that he needed. We spoke at length about chelation therapy, and he proceeded to telephone around the United States to doctors who administer it. Resnick affirms that he ran down every lead I had provided, and there were a lot of them.

Michael B. Schachter, M.D., gives the intravenous treatment, and Resnick took a two-hour drive twice weekly from West Hartford to the chelating doctor's office located in Nyack, New York, just over the Hudson River, crossing on the Tappan Zee Bridge.

"After taking three chelation treatments with Dr. Schachter, I found myself able to walk further and talk longer. After thirteen treatments, I told the young man who had been driving me that I didn't need him anymore. I drove myself for the four hours to and from Nyack. I remember that following my sixteenth treatment I attended a party in a friend's basement recreation room, and made innumerable trips up and down stairs without feeling any angina. I walked and talked with people non-stop. Those who had known how I had been feeling ill shortly before were amazed to see me so active," Resnick said.

"During the winter of that chelation therapy year, I was able to take long walks even in the coldest weather, and anginal pain never came on me. Without the need for nitroglycerine and Inderal, I could go on errands to the bank, post office, and shops," the patient continued. "I attribute this improvement to the benefits derived from taking chelation therapy.

"After having my thirtieth injection, a judgment was made by Dr. Schachter that I should take a break from chelation treatment for three months. I did this. Then, as a kind of insurance policy, I took another series of twelve intravenous injections in order to permanently get rid of the nitroglycerine and any other vasodilators I might have considered using," Resnick added.

The man continued to investigate alternatives even while undergoing chelation therapy and, as a friend, I suggested that he look into combining hyperbaric oxygen as an excellent adjunct to the intravenous treatment. After making his inquiries with various health authorities, he began a course of oxygen therapy in the hyperbaric chamber of Norwalk Hospital, Norwalk, Connecticut, under the supervision of Sreedhar Nair, M.D.

"I wasn't able to add hyperbaric oxygen until my twentieth chelation treatment. I took ten oxygen treatments in the morning on my way to receive my last ten chelation injections. This made for an extra long day: two hours driving down from Hartford with an hour and a half stop at Norwalk with Dr. Nair, four hours sitting in the lounge chair with my feet elevated taking the intravenous infusion under Dr. Schacter's supervision, and the two-hour drive home," Resnick explained. "The traveling caused me no trouble except for feeling slight fatigue at the end of the day."

Resnick is no longer considered in danger of a heart attack. When I visited with him recently at a Connecticut chapter meeting of the Association for Cardiovascular Therapies Inc., which I will describe in Chapter Seven, he looked to be in fine condition. Still, as an exponent of holistic health, the man continues to seek techniques for total fitness. He went on the stringent but full Pritikin program of diet and exercise. Now deceased, Nathan Pritikin, a Santa Monica, California, nutritionist, recommended eating a diet of just 10 percent fat, 10 percent protein, and 80 percent complex carbohydrates as one's daily food intake. No sugar or other refined carbohydrates are allowed in the diet. This eating program has proven itself advantageous for some people with cardiovascular disease and for those who want to avoid it.

Isadore Resnick said that he considers himself normal again. He experiences no more shortness of breath, no more chest pain, and for this interview he spoke to me about chelation therapy for several hours in an enthusiastic, animated way. The effort caused him no discomfort. "I'm really anxious for people to know the kinds of treatments available besides bypass surgery for heart patients," he said. "They must be informed about chelation therapy and other alternative methods of healing."

HOW CHELATION OCCURS

The medical specialty organization that certifies physicians as experts in administering chelation treatment, whose requirements I describe fully in Chapter Six, is called the American Board of Chelation Therapy (ABCT). ABCT defines chelation therapy as "a form of medical therapy designed to restore cellular homeostasis by the use of this metal binding and/or bio-inorganic agents. The proper application of this modality also requires knowledge of nutrition and exercise, as well as expertise in helping to implement other lifestyle changes."

Taken from the Greek word *chele* meaning "claw" (as the pincers of a crab or lobster), the term "chelation" refers to the way certain synthetic chemical and body proteins can bind metal molecules. The usual metal molecule possesses one, two, three, or more positive electrical charges. The chelating substance has extra negative charges that can combine with the positive ones of the metal and hold it fast in the clutching grip of the "claw" (*chele*). This gripping combination or "chelate" (see Figure 2.1 for a schematic drawing of a chelated molecule) takes on entirely different properties than the metal alone or the chelating substance alone. In effect, an entirely new and different chelated compound is formed whose atoms are firmly held together.

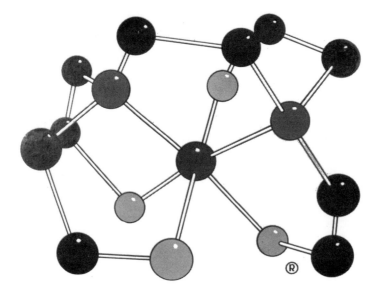

Figure 2.1. Schematic illustration of a mineral chelated with an amino acid.

The center mineral element is grasped by the bonds of the chelating substance and surrounded by it. Because the body does not have to make significant changes in the mineral ingested in this form, absorption and retention of this chelated mineral is very high. That is the chief advantage of consuming chelated minerals as dietary supplements.

The illustration from which this photograph was made was supplied through the courtesy of Albion Laboratories Inc.

The natural process of chelation is ongoing in the body. For instance, iron is a necessary metal present in your metabolic processes, and its transportation and migration in and out of your cells is handled by the chelation mechanism. This means that the dietary iron consumed in food is chelated within the tissues of your body.

Although tightly held in hemoglobin, which is the pigment present in red blood cells and the body's oxygen carrier, iron may be transported through the blood stream and dropped where it is needed in a tissue, organ, cell, or other part of the body. The binding of a metal such as iron is very sensitive to changes in body temperature, acidity, concentration of metal, concentration of chelating substance, presence of other metals, and the presence of other body chemicals. Such changes may bring about a release of iron and exchange it for another metal or for the binding of more or less iron molecules. In this way, the naturally present chelating substance hemoglobin can pick up iron and other metals from one location, transport them to another, and readily release them when the local tissue factors change.

A chelating protein made in the laboratory—a synthetic amino acid known to chemists as ethylene diamine tetraacetic acid (abbreviated EDTA)—acts in a way similar to hemoglobin. It binds with metals, locks them with its chelating pincers, and transports them out of the body. (See Figure 2.2 for a depiction of the actively working EDTA molecule.)

EDTA seems to work most effectively with metallic minerals that have two positive electrical charges. Lead, for example, contains two positive charges in its atomic ring, and EDTA combines with lead very well. For this reason, injecting EDTA into the body is the medically accepted and primary treatment for lead poisoning. Intravenous infusions with EDTA (chelation therapy) is the established method used around the world for the removal of heavy metals, such as mercury, cadmium, nickel, copper, lead, and others, from people who have toxic concentrations of these metals in their tissues.

Calcium, usually thought of as a mineral, has two positive charges in its ionic form, as well. This makes it capable of being chelated by EDTA, in the same way the reaction with lead takes place. Inject the appropriate strength and quantity of EDTA into a cardiovascular patient's blood vessels and calcium becomes tightly

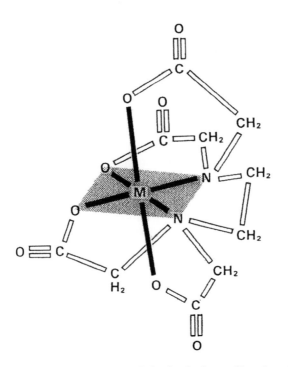

Figure 2.2.   Diagrammatic model of ethylene diamine tetraacetic acid (EDTA).

The "M" in the center area is a metal ion caught in a cagelike structure bound in place (chelated) by surrounding EDTA molecules. The dark lines depict EDTA bonds to the metal.

bound by it. The new chelated compound then gets excreted from the body through the kidneys and urinary tract as rapidly as the doctor determines, depending on how much and how fast he or she pours in the EDTA.

The same process goes on in the vegetable kingdom. A plant must have the mineral magnesium as part of its metabolic process in order to thrive. Chlorophyll, the green pigment that converts carbon dioxide and water into starch for the plant, is a chelator of magnesium. The plant uses chlorophyll for magnesium transport the same as your body uses hemoglobin for iron transport. Or, chlorophyll might be related to EDTA if a gardener injected chlorophyll into the plant for more effective magnesium transport the way a chelating physician injects EDTA for better calcium transport.

The amount of chelating EDTA and the rate at which it is given by the doctor must all be carefully controlled to avoid reactions and too rapid a reduction of blood calcium. Thirty years ago, in the United States, ethylene diamine tetraacetic acid was utilized in excessive quantities at too high a concentration in too short a period of infusion. The intravenous injection of EDTA for accomplishing chelation therapy received a bad press at that time. Two deaths occurred in 1954, the only two ever recorded from the administration of intravenous EDTA for the treatment of hardening of the arteries. Ever since then, chelation therapy has been living down the bad reputation it had acquired. Medical enemies of the treatment harp on those two old cases, which I discuss in Chapter Six, and repeat the liturgy of them over and over again. Chelation therapy opponents, either out of ignorance or maliciousness, fail to mention that over 500,000 Americans have been successfully treated with intravenous EDTA since 1954, with not one death occurring. And almost no side effects take place either.

Thus, the basic man-made amino acid used in chelation therapy, ethylene diamine tetraacetic acid, has the unique property of binding with divalent metals, including calcium, that have combined with cellular constituents in excess. Too much calcium is known to diminish the cellular enzyme function required to maintain viability in the arteries. When the EDTA is injected, it flushes the cells of ionic minerals, especially calcium, that are intricately woven with the various cell wall components and travels with them out of the body through the kidneys. To a lesser extent the solution and combined constituents go through the liver and thence are sent out through the gastrointestinal tract as waste products.

Testing reveals that a measurable and definite amount of ionized blood calcium is eliminated from the body this way. None of this is the calcium that has been bound in bones and teeth, but rather is metastatic or pathologic calcium causing damage to the body. It has been lightly bound to components within the arterial walls and even to the walls of the platelets and blood cells.

Thermograms, which are a diagnostic method showing heat pictures of body parts, taken before and after the chelation treatment, reveal that areas of impaired circulation frequently are restored to normal by this fascinating and efficient liquid engineer called EDTA.

THE ROLE OF CALCIUM IN ATHEROSCLEROSIS

Calcium is the most abundant mineral in the body. Of its total body content, 99 percent is lodged in the teeth and skeleton, and the balance makes up the soft tissue. To be metabolized for useful purposes, magnesium, phosphorus, and vitamins A, C, and D must be present in proper proportions.

The major function of calcium, most people know, is to build blood and maintain the bone structure. It also regulates the heart rate, assists in the process of blood clotting, prevents the accumulation of excess acid or alkali in the blood, eases insomnia, and must be present for muscle growth, muscle contraction, and the transference of nerve impulses. Without calcium, you would have an inability to utilize iron, you would be deficient in certain required body enzymes, and you would fail in your regulation of nutrient passage through the membranes of the approximately 80 trillion cells in your body.

Calcium can be a therapeutic element for the type of bone demineralization known as osteoporosis. Calcium ions floating freely in the blood—ionic calcium—stimulate hormones to bring minerals back to thinning bone structure. Phosphorus and magnesium enter into the reaction with calcium for this remineralization. Of the nutrients, calcium is the one that can help to overcome cramping feet and leg muscles. The restless legs syndrome experienced in bed at night by some people is aided by taking calcium supplementation. It has also been a protection source against sunburn, cancers caused by overexposure to radiation, bee stings, and is used to supply turgidity to cell walls for their transfer of fluids by osmotic pressure. In fact, calcium is a useful therapeutic agent in the following conditions: obesity, aging, gum disorders, acne, kidney dysfunction, mental illness, Parkinson's disease, Ménière's syndrome, rickets, colitis, fractures, celiac disease, constipation, worms, diabetes, anemia, pernicious anemia, and hemophilia.

The parathyroid glands, through their messenger hormone, parathormone, are the moderators of how much ionic calcium is permitted to be present in the blood. Furthermore, systemic calcium exists in several forms. In the teeth and bones, it is bound firmly to protein and other molecules and is not easily removed. In the blood it is also bound to protein, and to the other ionic form that I have mentioned, where the positive electrical charges are free to combine with negative charges present in additional blood substances.

The parathyroid glands carefully control the level of ionized calcium, for its variance beyond a narrow range can produce severe symptoms of discomfort and even death. But calcium storage in the body is rather inefficient, with just 25 percent being absorbed for physiological purposes. The unabsorbed calcium has two places to go: either as excrement in the feces or as metastatic calcium laid down where it does not belong. In other words, there are two forms of calcium, the appropriately absorbed and well-used ionic calcium and the poorly absorbed, distant spread of malignant calcium (known as calcium apatite).

Eating junk foods and a high-fat diet interfere with calcium absorption. The absorption process takes place in the duodenum and ceases in the lower part of the intestinal tract when the food content becomes alkaline. This most dominant mineral in the body needs acid for proper assimilation.

If acid fails to be present in a suitable amount, calcium won't dissolve and is rejected by the body as a precipitate. It doesn't go into ionic form for metabolic utilization. Instead, excessive calcium builds up in the tissues or joints as calcium deposits, leading to skin wrinkles, arthritis, hardening of the arteries, and other degenerative diseases.

It has been less than ten years now that the medical profession in the United States has recognized that calcium enters into the pathological process of coronary artery spasm and atherosclerotic plaque formation. On September 2, 1980, Richard Shanks interviewed me on his radio show, broadcasted from New Orleans, to explain the benefits of chelation therapy. In an equal time response demanded of radio station WWL by the Orleans Parish Medical Society, Richard Shanks then interviewed the designated representative of organized medicine named F. Filbert McMahon, M.D., four days later. In his interview, McMahon, clinical professor of medicine at Tulane University, past president of the American Society of Clinical Pharmacology and Therapeutics, and a member of the National Council on Drugs, erroneously said, "Hardening of the arteries isn't a disease of calcium . . . Removing the calcium from plaque by chipping it away has nothing to do with reversing the disease . . . Calcium is not present in atherosclerosis." Dr. McMahon is wrong! I possess a tape recording of the medical professor making those incorrect statements. The recording was sent to me by a New Orleans listener whose life had been saved by the use of chelation therapy.

Dr. McMahon's mistakes on that radio program are typical of the wrong thinking and misrepresentation of the truth made by agents of organized medicine as such errors related to chelation therapy. He broadcasted incorrect information to the millions of radio listeners around the southern states tuned into his rebuttal of my radio appearance. He implied that he intended to stop people from taking the treatment. In doing so, this physician, who presented himself as an authority on chelation therapy despite his admittedly never having given the treatment for heart disease or artery disease, may have prevented cardiovascular victims from extending their own lives. Surely the doctor must have persuaded some listeners when he said that chelation therapy "doesn't work."

In another misstatement, Dr. McMahon reported that the usual dose of intravenous EDTA was four grams. According to the protocol put forth by the true experts providing chelation therapy in the United States, physician members of the American College of Advancement in Medicine (ACAM), the four grams touted by this pharmacologist is an overdose. The ACAM considers three grams the maximum safe amount of EDTA to be administered at a single treatment. (See Chapter Six on safety and side effects.)

Then Dr. McMahon told Richard Shanks, "I was an expert witness here in federal court in New Orleans when a doctor in our community was giving it [intravenous EDTA]." What Dr. McMahon failed to mention is that H. Ray Evers, M.D., the chelating physician against whom Dr. McMahon had testified, sued this so-called expert witness for one million dollars in a libel action a year after the FDA case against Dr. Evers had been thrown out of court. The "expert" witness begged for an out-of-court settlement with Dr. Evers when he saw that the U.S. Justice Department would do nothing to defend him. It cost Dr. McMahon six thousand dollars of his own money and ten thousand dollars of his malpractice insurance company's money after Evers took pity on him and dropped the charges. The ten thousand dollars was paid to Dr. Evers on behalf of this medical professor who opposes chelation therapy. Dr. McMahon adhered to Dr. Evers' only other request that he issue a written apology for the libelous statements the defendant had made. Thus, on February 8, 1980, Dr. McMahon published a three-inch by two-inch notice in the *Montgomery Advertiser* and the *Atlanta Journal* retracting his misstatements. The only trouble is that misstatements about chelation therapy are seemingly still coming out of his mouth when he appears on the radio. This is an indication of how much representatives of establishment medicine know about chelation therapy and the way it works against calcium in atherosclerotic pathology.

Incidentally, the political power of organized medicine possibly is illustrated by what happened to program host Richard Shanks directly following the McMahon broadcast. Two days later, Richard Shanks was forced to leave radio station WWL. The dramatic change appeared mighty suspicious to thousands of Richard Shanks fans who faithfully tuned into his New Orleans talk show. Many listeners phoned me in outrage at the shabby treatment the radio host had received. The majority of listeners' opinions concluded that the station's management may have had pressure brought to bear by the local medical community, since Shanks had possibly been too supportive of a therapy that the Orleans Parish Medical Society did not favor.

In a more pleasant footnote, you should know that Shanks has gone on to excellent program-hosting positions first in Grand Rapids, Michigan, and now in Lakeland, Florida, at television station WTMV-TV (channel 32). Richard Shanks daily swallows quantities of oral chelating agents as a preventive against premature aging and to insure his good health. He is taking the oral chelates after checking with his physician, Donald J. Carrow, M.D., of Tampa, Florida, who provides his patients with chelation therapy. Shanks has again had proponents of chelation therapy as guests on his radio talk show. He has invited possible opponents to appear, but none would expose his or her own ignorance of the treatment to Shank's penetrating questions. He knows the facts!

Here are the scientific truths as they refer to whether calcium is or is not present in atherosclerotic plaque: "In atherosclerotic arteries there are marked changes in the structure of smooth muscle cells, elastic tissue, and in the internal lining as it relates to calcification," writes biotoxicologist Bruce W. Halstead, M.D., in his book, *The Scientific Basis of EDTA Chelation Therapy* (Golden Quill Publishers,

1979, hardcover). Dr. Halstead goes on to cite 1961 and 1964 re-search reports by Drs. L. E. Bolick and D.H. Blakenhorn showing two forms of calcifications occurring in blood vessels affected by cardiovascular disease. One form of calcification pathology "appears as discrete deposits of calcium" and the second form shows up "as a diffuse type involving primarily the elastic fibers of the arteries." Plaque in hardening of the arteries was analyzed by Dr. S. Y. Yu in 1974, and definitely consisted of calcium apatite along with many other materials. But calcium is the glue or binding substance that holds together all the junk material of atherosclerotic plaque.

THE FOUR TYPES OF HARDENING OF THE ARTERIES

Diseases of the arterial walls are classified into four distinct types: atherosclerosis, Mönckeberg's medial arteriosclerosis, hypertensive arteriosclerosis, and arteriolar sclerosis.

Atherosclerosis affects the internal wall of an artery. The central channel of the artery through which blood flows (the lumen) gets narrower until there is final and complete occlusion.

Mönckeberg's medial arteriosclerosis involves the arteries in the outer reaches of the body (the peripheral arteries), especially in the legs of middle-aged and older people. They form "pipestream arteries" from the deposition of calcium in their middle (medial) lining, but no disease encroachment occurs on the central tunnel through which blood flows.

Hypertensive arteriosclerosis is a progressive increase in muscle and elastic tissue of the arterial walls, resulting from chronic high blood pressure. In long-standing hypertension, elastic tissue forms numerous concentric layers on the inner arterial wall (the intima), and there is replacement of muscle tissue by connective tissue fibers. Degenerative thickening takes place. Such changes can develop with increasing age in the absence of hypertension and may then be referred to as **senile arteriosclerosis**. This is one of the underlying pathologies of senility.

Arteriolar sclerosis is a narrowing or closing of the tiniest of arteries that enter into the capillary network of the vascular tree.

Atherosclerosis is the artery and heart disease that is the most common and takes the largest number of lives. Every second person who dies in the United States each year has atherosclerosis as his or her cause of death. The disease slowly deteriorates the blood vessels throughout the entire arterial tree. Often its climax is a sudden and unexpected stroke or heart attack, but symptoms and signs will have appeared in other organs or regions of the body, which indicate that arteries in those locations are affected.

It is important for you to keep in mind that hardening of the arteries is not a localized or segmental disease; it does not affect only one part of the body at a time. Therefore, when Isadore Resnick underwent his coronary artery bypass operation, the surgeon wasn't doing much to overcome the patient's atherosclerosis. He was only bypassing approximately three inches of coronary artery clogged by atherosclerotic plaque. It was a heroic effort that served little purpose, for ten years later the bypass apparently, in a sudden occurrence, closed up altogether. Or a different segment in the same or another coronary artery became blocked with plaque. Resnick then had to look for a better, less life-threatening and less expensive technique to unclog the atherosclerosis. Chelation therapy offers that appropriate technique.

Remember, atherosclerosis is a "silent" disease that works its damage throughout the entire human organism and does not make itself known until it is almost too late to do much about it. Yet, almost every patient who has had a fatal heart attack was warned beforehand by some kind of symptom or sign. He may have had substernal chest pains (under the breast bone). He might have felt a tightness in the chest, a pain in the left jaw or aching of the left shoulder, or drawing and pulling sensations on the left side as though the individual had thrown an overly heavy object. Invariably there is some type of sign or symptom that strikes and gives a warning to the person. Usually one of these symptoms will hit the victim when he is under stress. Very few people die from hardening of the arteries without ever having received some precautionary signal beforehand.

CHAPTER THREE
How Chelating Agents Work in Your Body

A registered nurse, Eleanor Appleby of Irwin, Pennsylvania, described her experience having chelation therapy. Nurse Appleby wrote to me explaining, "At the age of 42, I sustained a very severe heart attack brought on by arteriosclerosis."

Like Isadore Resnick, the heart patient whose case I have described in Chapter Two, this woman underwent open heart surgery. Unfortunately, she experienced no particular change in the symptoms that had been present before the operation. The procedure turned out to be ineffective. She said that her chest pains continued. Dizzy spells came on her frequently and were really severe and frightening. Appleby accepted her condition for a while, realizing that she was gambling with fate. A fatal heart attack could strike her down at any time.

Awful angina remained without let-up and drove her to try something more. Nurse Appleby again undertook full physical and laboratory examinations and was told by the heart specialists that her arteries were so badly clogged that no more coronary artery bypass surgery was possible. They offered her nothing as an alternative and shrugged their collective shoulders with an implied, "I don't know what you're going to do now."

"The doctors literally sent me home to die," she wrote. Then she began putting her legal, social, and financial affairs in order so that there wouldn't be a burden on her loved ones at her passing.

As it happens, other nurse colleagues of Appleby's knew about chelation therapy and told her of a doctor in a southern state who provided the treatment at a hot mineral springs spa facility. She could become a resident of the health spa, take the mineral water baths and massages, the high colonic irrigations, and the detoxification techniques, and simultaneously enter the attached clinic as a chelation patient, also getting hyperbaric oxygen. Since this surely was her last resort to possibly find better health and life extension, Eleanor Appleby traveled south to receive five weeks of intravenous injections with a special chelating solution. The intravenous feedings were administered daily, three to four hours per injection.

"Before chelation therapy, walking just twenty-five feet had forced me to stop to catch my breath and rest so that I wouldn't fall over," Appleby said. "After only the third week of chelation therapy, I could walk miles without feeling any chest pain or dizziness."

When I visited Nurse Appleby's home area in Pittsburgh to gather chelation case histories and speak on chelation therapy to the Health Horizons Exposition, I saw that she looked exceedingly well. The grateful patient told me that she exercised daily by taking vigorous walks and hardly ever experienced angina. In addition to her nursing duties, she has taken on all the responsibility that goes with being the administrative secretary for a large non-profit organization. I checked out her medical history with many people who know her and found that what Eleanor Appleby had written to me was accurate and true.

This nurse had come under the care of H. Ray Evers, M.D., of Cottonwood, Alabama. Dr. Evers is the pioneering physician who has been repeatedly harassed by various agencies of the United States for giving his patients the intravenous chelation treatment that he has perfected and believes in. By denying him his civil rights guaranteed under the Constitution and available to every American, one governmental agency, the U.S. Food and Drug Administration, has designated Dr. Evers as the only practicing American physician not allowed to administer ethylene diamine tetraacetic acid in an intravenous infusion. Because he was denied the right to use EDTA chelation therapy to treat his patients, it became necessary for Dr. Evers to invent *Eversol*, another effective chelation solution.

Eversol consists of Ringer's lactate combined with various chelating (binding) agents, vitamins such as ascorbic acid, minerals such as magnesium and potassium, enzymes, and amino acids (which are administered all together intravenously to patients six or seven days a week). Just like EDTA, Eversol provides a recipient with chemo-endarterectomy, a non-surgical way of removing the plaque that forms inside his or her circulatory system.

HOW CHELATION REMOVES CALCIUM
AND OTHER METALS

Chelating solutions work in a bonding reaction, similar to a magnet attracting iron shavings.

Chemo-endarterectomy, or chelation (pronounced key-lay-shun), when administered as an infusion into the blood stream, acts to remove metals and metal compounds from the body, including but not limited to calcium. This was discussed in the previous chapter. The property of removing calcium from the areas in which it is deposited in the soft tissues of the body is vital because calcium is one of the most important substances present in the four types of arteriosclerosis, especially in the most common calcific atherosclerotic type that I have already explained. It binds together the coating of plaque that clogs the intimal and medial layers of the diseased blood vessels. This is established scientific fact; yet, we saw in Chapter Two that some physicians, in positions of great public responsibility and trust, incorrectly or falsely tell the public that calcium is an unimportant or negligible part of the symptomatic complex involving occlusive vascular disease.

When grossly misleading and outdated information is presented by the so-called orthodox medical establishment, disease and death are being foisted on medical consumers. This is severe and unfair punishment for patients who are relying on receiving true information in their attempts to determine their best course of action. Patients may decide to take vascular surgery and perhaps even have a fatal outcome, all based on lack of information or misstatements furnished by establishment physicians. And in some cases uneducated or dishonest practitioners of mainstream medicine are presenting wrong reports or innuendos simply because intravenous EDTA or other forms of chelation therapy are competing alternative methods of treatment to the surgery that these negligent doctors prefer to recommend.

The patient or his family may then learn that his physician's misrepresentation or omission is actually an act of medical malpractice under the *Cobbs v. Grant* legal doctrine of true and informed consent mandated by the law. Knowledge regarding the importance of calcium in cardiovascular disease has been extensively described throughout all of the latest scientific literature, including the official publications of the American Medical Association. There is no longer any excuse for a physician to hold back correct information regarding calcium antagonists and particularly chelation therapy from the patient who needs it. Failing to inform a patient about chelation therapy as a potential alternative to the usually recommended techniques of cardiovascular treatment could make the physician professionally liable for negligence in the performance of his duty.

The removal of calcium and other metals from the body by chelation solutions injected by chelating physicians is routinely substantiated by them with the use of chemical quantitative analyses of the chelated patients' urine. Urine excretion for each patient is gathered over a twenty-four-hour period for such an analysis.

WHERE THE METASTATIC CALCIUM COMES FROM

As calcium is removed from the blood by the chelating solution, it will be pulled out of other areas to keep the calcium blood level constant. The readily available areas to supply this need are the deposits of metastatic calcium spread around the body in wrinkled skin, arthritic joints, kidney stones, and calcified bursae, which often produce symptoms of bursitis. But of all the sources of metastatic calcium (calcium apatite) that serve to replace the missing serum ionic calcium, it is the calcium apatite present in the walls of clogged arteries that surrender the most.

Thus, those hot spots in the body where calcium has been abnormally laid down as dregs, and where it is loosely bound, supply the new calcium atoms required to go into solution in the blood as ionized calcium. This is the physiological basis for how injected or ingested chelating agents work in the body to provide you with a chemo-endarterectomy effect.

Take a chelating agent into your body, and some calcium detritus will come off the inner walls of your blood vessels, from around tendons, joints, ligaments, the skin, kidneys, pancreas, and other places that have precipitated calcium to get rid of. In this way abnormal calcium deposits or calcifications can be gradually reduced over a period of time because of the unique properties of chelating substances. (See Figures 3.1 and 3.2, showing calcium deposits removed from the skin by the use of EDTA.)

Unquestionably calcium apatite is not the only bad stuff making up atherosclerotic plaque, but it does act as a mucilaginous material—the cementing substance—that binds together much of the clogging junk. When metastatic calcium is chelated out of plaque and off the diseased blood vessel walls, the remaining bad stuff containing fatty globules, cholesterol, mucopolysaccharides, fibrin, collagen, foreign proteins, various minerals, blood elements, and such other material floating in the path of the plaque tend to sepa-

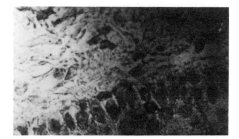 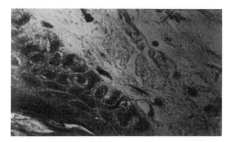

1. Taken before chelation therapy, the subcutaneous, or fatty muscular layer that lies below the skin, is shown at the upper portion of the photograph, while the larger, well-demarcated darker cells that make up the cutaneous, or skin layer, is at the lower portion of this photograph.

2. The same skin areas are depicted after they have received chelation therapy. Note that the metastatic calcium is much less in the loosely bound, relatively non-cellular areas of the upper portions of this photograph. This indicates that EDTA has removed the excessive calcium from the skin. Compare the two photographs; the heavier, coarser, and more granular material from 1 has diminished in 2.

Figure 3.1.　Microphotographs of skin depicting calcium deposits, before and after chelation therapy.

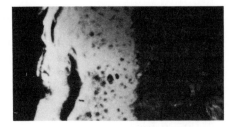 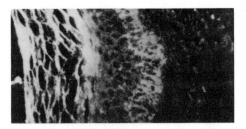

1. A biopsy slice through the skin is depicted here, with the dark area at the left being the outer skin layer. The white and milky materials shown here are the fatty deposits present before chelation therapy.

2. The same biopsied skin area is shown after chelation therapy has been received by the patient. Note that the concentration of white fatty deposits have been greatly reduced. By reducing the calcium content through intravenous EDTA, the health status of the skin is increased as well. This microphotograph shows the skin's improved health.

Figure 3.2.   Microphotographs of skin depicting fatty acids, before and after chelation therapy.

rate. The plaque gets mushy and can better be absorbed or removed by the cleansing action of the blood.

With a chelating agent floating through your blood stream bringing about this effect, the advantage to you is that the lumen or open portion of the narrowed blood vessel then becomes wider. More blood can flow through it to the cells, tissues, organs, or parts that are showing signs of distress. Function improves.

Even an extremely small increase in the diameter of the blood vessel's lumen will heighten the flow through it by a much greater proportion. For instance, an increase in one millimeter in diameter of the lumen will permit a four-fold increase in blood flow. This greater circulatory capacity is the vital factor for cells, tissues, organs, body parts, and whole body systems.

In summary, by injecting a synthetic amino acid such as EDTA, a chelating natural substance like vitamin C, or a combination of perhaps a dozen other ingredients similar to the Eversol formula developed by Dr. H. Ray Evers, all that the doctor is doing is copying Nature's technique of handling metallic minerals. It is an extremely valuable method that is being furnished to patients by courageous physicians who are bucking the medical establishment at personal costs to their careers, respectability, prestige, and other distinctions that accompany being a member of the healing professions. (See the medical politics in Chapter Seven.)

Chelation therapy has been devised to safely counteract directly the harmful effects of calcium deposits in the circulatory system. Traditional physicians who don't know this may become the enemies of chelation treatment. Those physicians who witness the procedure's benefits for their patients soon turn into the newest chelation mavericks in medicine, unless they have some vested interest in ignoring how the chelating agent works. Who would be these narrow-minded boneheads with vested interests to protect? Perhaps heart surgeons, peripheral vascular surgeons, chest surgeons, some cardiologists who receive high remuneration for post-coronary patient care, and others of that type.

When combined with a proper nutritional program of live balanced foods, the use of vitamin and mineral supplements in the proper amounts, the daily ingestion of oral chelating agents, an anti-stress program to combat various disease factors in our environment, and an appointed routine of therapeutic exercises such as jogging, swimming, calisthenics, rebounding, skipping rope, cycling, rowing, or another activity of an aerobic nature, chelation therapy helps to reverse hardening of the arteries. The results reported by almost five thousand chelated people whom I have interviewed during the twelve years of my involvement with this treatment, especially those following up with the lifestyle I am suggesting, have been almost miraculous.

The excellent healing power of chelation therapy produces marked improvement in circulatory function by restoring a new elasticity to the blood vessel walls. If you, too, make the attempt to remove the detritus of metastatic calcium from the arterial intima and media, you will find that hardening of your arteries goes away. You're able to do this with various types of chelating agents. EDTA received by injection isn't the only way to unharden your arteries.

VARIOUS TYPES OF CHELATING AGENTS

Aspirin is a chelating agent. Aspirin chelates away the anti-endorphin factor that gets trapped in the pain gate present in the brain that makes your head hurt. Citric acid and other weak organic acids, such as ascorbic acid, lactic acid, and acetic acid, are also chelating agents. In fact, lactic acid produced by your own muscles when you exercise is an excellent way to clean the metastatic calcium off your arterial walls or out of your arthritic joints. The formation of natural chelating lactic acid is another good reason, besides the aerobic strengthening of your heart, to exercise routinely at a regularly appointed time each day.

Other common pharmaceutical agents that work, at least partially, through the chelation mechanism are cortisone, Terramycin™, and adrenaline. A host of chelating compounds, natural and synthetic, exist—probably numbering in the tens of thousands. In Part Two, I will describe lots of oral chelating agents, acquired either through direct purchase in a foreign country, over-the-counter in this country, by mail order, by doctor's prescription, or directly from your doctor, that you can employ yourself at home for unhardening your arteries. I must include a word of caution right away; however, oral chelating agents work best as a preventive measure against occlusive vascular disease. If you are well, oral chelators can be counted on to keep you that way. If you have signs or symptoms of hardening of the arteries, oral chelating agents are not enough to get you well. They work too slowly by themselves. Intravenous (IV) EDTA chelation therapy works best for the fast remedy often required to overcome occlusive vascular illness. Intravenous (IV) chelation therapy must be administered, of course, under the supervision of a trained specialist in the treatment. He or she will likely provide you with prescribed oral chelating nutrients or pharmaceuticals to accompany the infusions you get. Depend on the ACAM-trained physician to combine oral and intravenous chelation therapy.

Mineral therapy and vitamin therapy are integral additions to the EDTA chelation injection treatment. Many vitamins and minerals are themselves oral chelating agents. Soviet physicians employ a chelator called *Unithiol*™ with a multivitamin administration for the treatment of coronary arteriosclerosis. The Russians encourage the use of vitamin and mineral supplements for their population. Soviet medical scientists have concluded that early treatment with dietary supplements and chelation injections provides the most successful approach against coronary artery disease and heart disease. They recommend this combination for the prevention of hardening of the arteries and premature aging. The protocol of the American College of Advancement in Medicine Inc. makes this recommendation, as well.

Unithiol™ employs a sulfhydryl group in its molecular makeup. Sulfhydryl is a chelator. When combined with orthomolecular nutrition, which uses megadose nutritional supplements, and regular exercise, the Soviet physicians find the approach so successful that some knowledgeable Russian doctors now use it for their patients and themselves as an anti-aging procedure. Orthomolecular nutrition, routine exercise, and chelation therapy turn back the clock on the wearing out of cells to reduce the incidence of hardening of the arteries for many older people. A similar program is provided for the populace of Czechoslovakia. In these two countries, Russia and Czechoslovakia, chelation therapy is the most commonly used treatment against all kinds of degenerative diseases derived from hardening of the arteries.

Another, supposedly better intravenous amino acid substance exists besides EDTA. EGTA or ethyl-glycol-bis-beta-amine-ethyl-ether-N, N-tetraacetic acid is a chelating substance that avoids the production of any free radical effect, particularly when it is mixed in even minute portions with copper or iron. A free radical is an atom or molecule that possesses at least one unpaired electron which does great damage in cells or tissues by colliding with other free radicals to set up a chain reaction.

DMSO or dimethyl sulfoxide also acts as a chelating agent when administered intravenously, consumed as a drink, or rubbed on the skin. One of DMSO's derivatives, methylsulfonylmethane (MSM), is an oral chelator that I describe at length in Part Two.

A world authority on molecular oxygen and free radical damage, Harry B. Demopoulos, M.D., who is chief pathologist at New York University Heights College, told the Tenth Anniversary Spring Conference of the American College of Advancement in Medicine, held in Los Angeles May 20-22, 1983, that the nutrients citric acid, glycine (an amino acid), gluconic acid, and histidine (another amino acid) are low-toxicity chelating agents that work well by intravenous injection.

Cystine, glutathione reductase, and methionine are also good heavy-metal binders, although they are not without side effects. Methionine use, for instance, must be matched with vitamin B-6 supplementation. Eskimos sustaining themselves on a raw-meat diet are a population relatively free of cardiovascular disease, despite their high fat intake. Why? Raw meat has sufficient vitamin B-6 to handle methionine problems. When meat is cooked, this natural balance is phased out and cardiovascular disease occurs among populations that make such a dietary change.

Your body's cells are exquisitely sensitive to damage from free radical proliferation that comes from exposure to stress such as sunburn, environmental temperature changes, food additives, cigarette smoke, lack of exercise, fatigue, emotional upset, physical injury, and other traumas. Peroxidation occurs, which is a splitting off of hydrogen atoms in various body substances, and this leads to atherosclerosis, most malignancies, senescence, and much inflammatory disease. The cellular membrane damage caused by free radicals, especially when your body's three main anti-free radical-scavenging enzyme systems are depressed or absent, directly sets the stage for cancer, says Dr. Demopoulos. The enzymes that fight off free radicals are the superoxide dismutase system, the catalase system, and glutathione peroxidase.

Peroxidation of cellular membranes allows calcium to be "pumped into the cell hence causing many other damaging reactions," Dr. Demopoulos affirms, and this helps to predispose you to the formation of hardening of the arteries. What's the solution to preventing this blood vessel breakdown? Take oral chelating agents on a prevention basis such a vitamins A, C, and E, certain amino acids, tripeptides, certain steroids, the hormone DHEA, and a few estrogen-related compounds. But only take these chelating compounds under a chelation physician's supervision. They are effective antioxidants and therefore anti-free radical components needed by the body, says the pathologist. A really good oral chelator is aspartic acid, which is discussed in Part Two.

LACK OF PROMOTION OF CHELATION THERAPY

Why isn't chelation treatment generally employed in American medicine? In the political report that I present in Chapter Seven, you will learn about aspects of medicine that are buried under the proverbial rug. For now you should be made aware that one reason chelation therapy isn't generally accepted by practicing physicians lies in the lack of promotion being given the treatment by pharmaceutical companies. Organized medicine and the pharmaceutical industry seem to lie comfortably in bed together for the winning of consumers' dollars.

There isn't much money in pushing the use of chelation therapy by organized medicine for large pharmaceutical companies because the patent ran out on EDTA in 1948. Drug firms could not protect their financial investment in promoting the intravenous use of EDTA. Even if some industry executives were inclined to make that magnanimous investment for the singular reason that chelation therapy saves lives, it's likely that company stockholders would veto such a decision.

With no multimillion-dollar campaign going to advertise it to the medical profession, doctors are disinclined to prescribe chelation therapy. Some actually don't know that it exists. Others are predisposed to prescribe only what is a popular drug at the time. Inasmuch as the EDTA material has been available too long and can't be patented, no large pharmaceutical company is even anxious to produce it. There isn't much profit to be made.

Unfortunately, in our society great ideas often lay dormant if there is no promotional push to let everyone know about it. Certainly few laypersons know that chelation therapy is available. Your reading of this book may be the first time you are exposed to the full story of this excellent treatment, which has been accessible to your physician in this country since 1948.

Because pharmaceutical companies and the government are the only institutions able to afford the large expenditures necessary to bring chelation therapy to the attention of the medical profession so that doctors, in turn, may advise the public, it's no wonder that nothing much has been heard about the treatment. A tremendous amount of research and promotion are required to market a drug for the specific purposes recommended for it in this book.

The good news is that there are many studies presently going on at clinics, doctors' offices, and universities to find out more about how these amazing chelating materials work both inside and out of the body. In Chapter Five, I will shed some light on a few of those studies. Not publicizing clinical studies until now has also been a source of contention on chelation therapy between traditionalists and mavericks in medicine. You will learn in Chapter Seven why, in 1963, intravenous chelation therapy got a black eye from the publication of just one slightly negative paper and how, in 1968, research had been discontinued on the use of intravenous EDTA. Then, in 1981 it finally began again.

But more and more physicians are turning to the use of chelating materials. They are the best means to help victims of vascular disease, primarily because there is little else to offer these patients. Surgery is proving useful only as an emergency stop-gap, since cardiovascular disease doesn't affect just segments of the system but attacks the entire vascular tree at once. The disease continues on following the segmental surgery. And dietary improvement is only part of the answer. Performing routine exercise, cutting out smoking, and taking all the drugs now on the market doesn't even seem to do much to discourage the deposits of plaque from forming in the arteries.

CHELATION TREATMENT FOR LEAD POISONING

Chelation agents are somewhat like aspirin in that all of the mechanisms by which they exert their beneficial effects are presently still not known. Moreover, practically every enzyme in your body has some small amount of metal involved in its chemical structure. Such a metal is bound in chelated form. Without certain trace metals, the particular enzyme that is missing then becomes inactive and does you no good.

On the other hand, too much of the heavy metals may replace the normal mineral content of metabolic enzymes. The enzyme protein structure becomes divergent and blocks the proper enzyme action desired by the body. Then you will feel a variety of symptoms, because you can get in trouble with organ dysfunction. This is how excess lead, mercury, antimony, arsenic, aluminum, copper, nickel, cadmium, and other environmental metallic poisons may damage vital internal structures. The heavy minerals block normal enzymes and prevent their metabolic activity. Heavy metals work over a long period to damage and destroy, sometimes causing the uninformed doctor to make an erroneous diagnosis. The unknowing physician may come up with virus infection, "old age," neurosis, psychosomatic or some other label he or she invents as the substitute for a condition that he or she fails to understand.

Something of this nature happened to Philip Lee, the father of Eugene H. Lee, M.D., a general medical practitioner specializing in acupuncture, who is located in Tampa, Florida. Dr. Lee, 43 years old, has taken chelation therapy for thirty-three treatments during the past year to prevent any possible cardiovascular diseases. "I do my nutrition and exercise program faithfully," he writes. "I want to keep my good health and also prove to my patients that the chelation therapy program works. I have been administering chelation therapy for six years."

Philip Lee lives in Taiwan. He was feeling poorly and didn't know why. Visits that he made to his doctors on the distant island never availed him much relief. Lucky for Mr. Lee that he now has a son who is a holistic physician practicing in the United States.

As a result of the encouraging developments in the increased health of his patients by following the precepts of holistic medicine advocated by Dr. Lee, he wanted to do the same thing for his parents. Therefore, a few years ago he asked his father to send a hair sample for testing. Dr. Lee's intent was to check Philip Lee's tissue content for heavy metals overload or essential minerals deficiency that the man's hair mineral analysis might possibly reveal.

"Surprisingly, my father's head hair showed a lead level of 668 parts per million [ppm]," said Dr. Lee. This is an exceedingly elevated level of lead in the human body and usually leads to severe disease symptoms. The highest level of lead considered safe for a person is 15 ppm. Anything over 100 ppm could be diagnosed as lead poisoning.

"Alarmed, I telephoned him overseas immediately," Dr. Lee continued. "It was then that he revealed his use of a hair preparation called Youth Hair, to darken his hair; otherwise, it would show its naturally greying color. He had purchased the hair preparation in a New York City department store during his last visit to America, about four years ago. As soon as I realized the potential health hazard of his using this hair dye, I asked him to discontinue its application and to send a pubic hair sample as a replacement. This time his pubic hair mineral analysis showed a tissue lead level of 344 ppm. My dad was absorbing excessive quantities of lead from the head hair preparation. Checking the label on a bottle of Youth Hair, I saw that its content of lead acetate is printed at the corner in very small letters, trying to avoid people's attention."

Through a series of letters and telephone calls, Dr. Lee prevailed upon his father to come to the United States to take chelation therapy in order to remove the accumulated lead from his body. Finally Philip Lee adhered to his son's advice.

"When he arrived in this country, my dad complained about feeling lethargic, with general weakness, tennis elbow, loss of memory, and some other problems. He had been experiencing these symptoms for the past several months, possibly from the built-up quantity of lead that was poisoning his body," said the physician.

Additional signs and symptoms of lead toxicity a person could exhibit include headache, depression, insomnia and/or drowsiness, fatigue, nervousness, irritability, dizziness, confusion and disorientation, anxiety, muscle wasting, muscle aching, saturnine gout, abdominal pain, loss of appetite, loss of weight, constipation, hypertension, defective kidneys, decreased fertility in men, spontaneous abortion in women, impaired adrenal function, iron deficiency anemia, and blue-black lead lines near the base of the teeth.

"After I gave my father thirty chelation treatments, all of his symptoms of lead poisoning were gone. He told me that he felt wonderful and this special trip to the United States for taking chelation was as worthy as winning a million U.S. dollars. He has now gone back to Taiwan," Dr. Lee said. "From his correspondence, I see that my father is following my instructions, taking vitamin and mineral supplements and other oral chelating agents, doing regular exercises, and avoiding the drinking of coffee and liquor completely. Of course he isn't using any hair preparation and does not care anymore if his hair color turns grey."

Not only had Philip Lee been exposed to lead poisoning, but his wife Nancy also showed a lead level of 43 ppm in her head hair, although she had never used head preparations. Dr. Lee wrote: "My mother Nancy Lee also took 36 chelation treatments when she was visiting me with my father. She had several years history of arthritis and hypertension, but after chelation therapy she is back to her regular activity and feels much younger and more energetic. As a matter of fact, she passed her driver's license examination at the age of 62."

A year after the initial hair mineral testing of his parents, Dr. Eugene Lee found that his mother's head hair reading remained at 13 and that his father's stayed at 24.

The absorption of lead and the deposition of calcium in abnormal locations are continuous throughout life so that true preventive therapy should involve chelating them out at regular intervals to prevent too great a build up in the arteries and other tissues. It may eventually be necessary for survival for our next generation to require periodic chelation treatment to delead their bodies. Children are more at risk than anyone else.

The potential long-term effects of lead exposure are just beginning to be realized when it is appreciated that children are getting huge quantities into their bodies by just playing in dirt or dust that is constantly exposed to the fallout from smog or winds carrying exhaust fumes from the nation's highways and freeways. On August 26, 1983, the United States Court of Appeals in Washington, D.C., ruled that the Department of Housing and Urban Development had failed in its duty to protect children from the poisonous effects of lead-based paint.

The court said that under a 1973 law, the agency was required to "establish procedures to eliminate as far as practicable the hazards of lead-based-paint poisoning" in any property owned or subsidized by the federal government. But the department had failed to do so. Instead, the department had narrowly construed its obligations according to a cost-benefit analysis for which there was no legal justification. The court had ruled on a case filed in 1981 on behalf of public housing tenants in the District of Columbia, but the decision has nationwide implications for the 2.8 million families who receive federal housing assistance.

"Congress was intensely concerned with public health menace of lead poisoning and clearly intended to bring the power of the federal government to bear in ameliorating the problem," the appeals court said. "Lead poisoning, the accumulation of lead in body tissues, is a serious health problem, particularly for children. Lead

poisoning in children may affect the central nervous system, causing convulsions, coma and permanent brain damage or death. Approximately 200 children in the United States die each year from
lead poisoning, and as many as 10,000 additional children suffer
significant adverse effects from the condition."

Children swallow the poisonous lead when they eat chips or
flakes of lead-based paint and when they chew on painted surfaces,
such as window sills and door frames. Although the sale of lead-
based paint has been banned for two decades, the danger lies with
old lead-based painted surfaces covered over with new unleaded
paint that has chipped away, exposing the old lead-based painted
surface.

A federal study completed in 1982 revealed that one of every
twenty-five preschool children had an unacceptably high level of
lead in his blood. The problem was found to persist in middle-class
suburban neighborhoods as well as inner-city poor neighborhoods.
The only way that lead is effectively removed from the child's body
is by chelation therapy with ethylene diamine tetraacetic acid. Over
200,000 American children have received the treatment in which
EDTA combines with blood lead and is excreted. If chelation therapy is safe enough to use on children, even youngsters eighteen
months old, as is common in the lead belts around the United
States such as in the Bedford-Stuyvesant housing development in
New York City, why isn't the treatment safe enough to remove
metastatic calcium from the bodies of adults? Well, it is! Chelation
therapy reverses pathology in degenerative diseases when the pathology arises from blood vessel occlusion, heavy mineral toxicity,
especially involving calcium, and arterial wall spasm from excessive
calcium concentration. You will be made aware of the conditions
corrected with chelation treatment when you read about them in
the next chapter.

CHAPTER FOUR
Corrective Uses of Chelation Therapy

The man had a problem shared by one out of ten adult American males. It was a problem that he wouldn't discuss with his family physician or even his wife, although the couple in their loving relationship were conscious of being its victims. He had felt overwhelmed. He knew it was affecting his self-image. His wife wanted to know what caused his problem and whether there was a cure.

The problem was impotence. In a city the size of Los Angeles, sex counselors estimate that more than 100,000 men suffer from impotence (referred to medically as "erectile difficulty"). Ten million Americans are permanent victims of erectile difficulty, and approximately 50 percent of the other men have potency problems more than just occasionally.

Erectile difficulty is defined as the inability to achieve or maintain an erection satisfactory for sexual intercourse. This problem afflicts men of all ages, and it is devastating to them and their partners. As one of its victims explained, "It makes you feel like a failure, not just in your sex life, but in other situations as well. You lose confidence in yourself."

Therapists report that depression, guilt, and anger often accompany impotence, and a woman attached to the man experiencing such difficulty may also share these feelings. Until very recently, medical experts believed that the causes of impotence were largely psychological. Men bold enough to seek professional help were most often told, "It's all in your head; relax and forget about it," or were referred to sex therapy. Results varied greatly but mostly ended in failure.

Recently it has been established that there has been an overemphasis on mental aspects of getting and holding an erection. While it is true that you can lose an erection if you believe you will, the physical aspects have too often been overlooked. Now, medical experts understand that as many as half of the cases of erectile difficulty are due to physical, and frequently treatable, causes. Erectile difficulty may indicate blocked arteries to the male genitals.

Trouble with erectile response ultimately occurs in almost 50 percent of the adult males with diabetes. Vascular problems such as high blood pressure and the drugs taken to lower one's blood pressure can cause the problem. Other causes include hormonal disorders, spinal cord injury, cancer surgery, alcoholism, drug abuse, multiple sclerosis, Parkinson's disease, and a host of other lesser health problems such as mineral imbalance, allergy, subclinical illness, and upper respiratory congestion. Determining whether impotence is physical or psychological is the important first step in getting rid of such a problem.

This was what 56-year-old Beuford Masterson, a tobacco farmer living on the outskirts of Kingston, Tennessee, finally came to do. Because his penis would not respond to the sexual demands of his young wife, their marriage was deteriorating. The woman declared that she loved him, but her urges for sex required fulfillment. She felt frustrated and angry. The ultimatum this man's wife eventually levied forced Beuford to finally seek medical attention.

Donald C. Thompson, M.D., D.Ph. of Morristown, Tennessee, who is a faculty member in the Department of Medicine of Meharry Medical College, School of Medicine, diagnosed Masterson as the victim of Leriche syndrome. Leriche syndrome consists of gradual occlusion of the lowest portion of the aorta where it divides into the two arteries sending blood to the right and left halves of the body. And the patient's impotence was a secondary symptom to his main health problem, which was peripheral vascular disease in his lower extremities.

It was with this diagnosis that Masterson faced reality and acknowledged that for years he had been feeling closer and closer intervals of pain in the calves when he attempted to climb stairs or to work his tobacco fields. He had reached the point of being able to walk only 200 feet when the pain in his calf muscles came on so unrelentingly, the man had to stop dead in his tracks until the pain passed. It was taking him about four minutes to walk the equivalent of just one long city block.

As it happened, the condition of intermittent claudication was affecting both of Masterson's legs and his penis, as well. Intermittent claudication is a cramping pain, induced by exercise and relieved by rest, that comes from an inadequate supply of blood to the affected muscles. It is most often seen in the calf and leg muscles as a result of blood clots and narrowing of the leg arteries. The leg pulses are often absent and the feet may feel cold or be cold to touching fingers.

For Masterson, claudication in the calves was due to narrowing of the femoral arteries and their branches; gangrene of the toes was a very real possibility for the man. While gangrene of the penis rarely happens, his manifestation of claudication in that organ took the form of his never getting an erection anymore.

Men joke about the penis and sometimes call it their "love muscle." But it isn't really a muscle so much as it is a tube (the urethra) surrounded by spongy tissue and some muscles. It is the spongy tissue that firms up by filling with blood when aroused. When erect, the penis will grow two and a half times its usual thickness and fill with 200 times its usual volume of blood. If arteries are blocked in the genital area, an erection won't be as firm as normal, or won't occur at all.

Sheldon O. Burman, M.D., medical director of the Male Sexual Dysfunction Institute in Chicago, reported to the American College of Advancement in Medicine during its May 1983 scientific conference, held in Los Angeles, that blood flow in the penis is quite measurable. Dr. Burman employs newer diagnostic techniques and has observed that many patients with erectile impotence have inadequate blood flow to the penis because of arteriosclerosis of its arteries.

"We use a special instrument cuff to record the penile pulse volume and blood pressure," said Dr. Burman. "As a man gets older, vascular constriction is the most probable reason for erectile difficulties. We can reproduce the phenomenon of erection in the impotent male by putting the reduced-size blood pressure cuff on the base of the penis, inflating the cuff, eliminating the pulse, leaving the inflated cuff in place for a few minutes, and with releasing the pressure, a normal hyperemic response takes place. It is like stuffing blood into the organ [which expands as if the man acquired his usual erection from a sexual stimulus]. This helps the doctor determine the response of the penis to blood supply deprivation or, to put it another way, he can stimulate what normally occurs with his patient's erection."

Riding the crest of what he calls a "remarkable growing field," Barton Bean, director of non-invasive vascular laboratory medicine at the University of Arizona Health Sciences Center and the Veterans Administration Hospital in Tucson, Arizona, also pointed out at the Tenth Anniversary Spring 1983 Conference of ACAM that "the use of the penile blood pressure cuff, either for taking blood pressures or doing plethysmography, is becoming a standard in the health industry for impotence studies." Penile blood pressure is known to go way down when erectile difficulties from occlusive vascular diseases are present.

For more information about this impotency diagnostic technique and the program for correcting male sexual dysfunction, contact Sheldon O. Burman, M.D., Male Sexual Dysfunction Institute, 3401 North Central Avenue, Chicago, Illinois 60634, telephone (312) 725-7722. You can also contact the American International Clinic, telephone (800) 367-4357 or the Non-invasive Vascular Laboratory at the University of Arizona College of Medicine, telephone (602) 882-6214.

The American International Clinic in Zion, Illinois, uses chelation therapy as one of the major modalities for the correction of erectile difficulty due to the blockage of blood supply to the penis. And this treatment is what Dr. Thompson employed to correct Beuford Masterson's Leriche syndrome.

The patient was begun at first only on oral chelating agents in April 1980, instead of subjecting him to the long automobile ride to Morristown from his farm in Kingston to take intravenous injections with EDTA. Masterson continued on the oral supplementation program for one year, during which time his exercise tolerance improved from 200 feet to being able to walk 300 yards before needing a rest from the pain in his calf muscles. His Leriche syndrome remained unchanged, however, a situation about which he and his wife were disappointed.

Mrs. Masterson exhibited patience with her husband's continued inability to satisfy her sexually, inasmuch as the man was attempting to remedy his condition under medical supervision. She made sure that he faithfully took the oral chelating agents dispensed by Dr. Thompson.

His physician discussed the procedure of EDTA chelation therapy with his patient and then cautiously started him on a course of treatment. It began slowly in April 1981 with just one intravenous infusion at a frequency of every three to six weeks. By the time Masterson had received five treatments, he reported improvement in his ability to walk better than a quarter of a mile before having to stop for calf-pain relief. More than this, the man joyously told of his being able to fulfill his wife's needs at least twice with "good, vigorous erections." They had allowed for truly satisfying sexual intercourse for both of them.

Since then Masterson has continued with intravenous chelation injections and his oral chelating agents so that by July 1, 1983, the date I received this case history, he had taken thirty-six treatments. The man advised Dr. Thompson that his sex life is superb. He can get an erection and engage in sexual activity any time the urge mutually comes upon him and his mate. In fact, Masterson said that his wife was beginning to complain about the lack of sleep she was getting. The farmer also reports virtually no exercise limitation. He finds himself able to tramp over acres of tobacco fields without any need to stop due to pain. Intermittent claudication of the calves and erectile difficulty are gone altogether as a result of his oral and intravenous chelation therapy.

OTHER CONDITIONS CORRECTED BY CHELATION

A variety of chelating agents have been utilized for a diverse number of therapeutic purposes. Of the many agents available, ethylene diamine tetraacetic acid has provided by far the best remedial effects in degenerative diseases for patients of all ages; therefore, EDTA is the chelator I will be speaking about in this section on conditions benefited by chelation therapy.

Chelation treatment has been successfully applied in heavy metal poisoning and atherosclerosis, as already discussed, but it also has found usefulness in the following conditions: myocardial and coronary insufficiency, cerebral arteriosclerosis, Alzheimer's disease, senile dementia, schizophrenia, rheumatoid arthritis, osteoarthritis, gouty arthritis, calcific tendonitis, calcific bursitis, kidney stones, gallbladder stones, multiple sclerosis, lupus erythematosus, Parkinson's disease, Lou Gehrig's disease, cataracts, glaucoma, cancer, osteoporosis, varicose veins, hypertension, scleroderma, Raynaud's disease, digitalis intoxication, heart arrhythmias, hypercalcemia, heart valve calcification, peripheral vascular insufficiency, intermittent claudication, aortic calcinosis, aneurysm, cerebral ischemia, stroke, diabetes, diabetic ulcers, diabetic gangrene, diabetic retinopathy, macular degeneration, emphysema, leg ulcers, venomous snake bite, and any other condition where the problem is an interruption in blood flow because of atherosclerotic plaque, arterial spasm due to excessive calcium ion concentration, a sluggishness of the parathyroid glands in calcium metabolism, or a lack of collateral circulation.

Because so many conditions are correctable with chelation therapy and their improvements are based on similar physiological changes in pathology, I will briefly discuss just a few of the more common degenerative diseases affecting people in Western industrialized society that are aided by the treatment. The conditions relating to blood flow impairment to be described include diabetes, gallstones, kidney diseases from poor circulation, stroke, emphysema, cataracts, senility, macular degeneration, varicose veins, Parkinson's disease, osteoporosis, a bone disorder called Paget's disease, and hypertension.

Of every hundred Western people around the world between ages 18 and 80 today, cardiovascular specialists advise that fourteen have definite heart disease and twelve more probably do. Furthermore, of the ten biggest killers of Americans (in the order of their frequency) including heart disease, cancer, stroke, accidents, pneumonia, diabetes, cirrhosis, arteriosclerosis, suicides, and infant death, all but accidents, pneumonia, suicides, and infant death have an underlying connection to diminishing of the blood circulation.

Ninety-five percent of us live in jeopardy of having a serious illness relating to the circulatory system. Besides the six killer diseases out of the ten major conditions causing death in industrialized Western countries indicated in the listing just given, others that have a blood constriction precursor are digestive problems, arthritis, hypertension, parkinsonism, psoriasis, muscular dystrophy, leg ulcers, and many more afflictions. These conditions occur from hindered circulation of the blood to vital organs. The cells of these organs fail to receive constantly required essential nutrients. Also they lack the removal of toxic residues of metabolism. Any interference with the free flow of blood upsets the functioning of cells and causes them to cease resisting poisons, which will ultimately bring on organ or tissue disease.

Degenerative Diseases Lacking Free Blood Flow

Particular diseases come from deterioration and loss of the specialized function of the cells of a tissue or organ and subsequently bring about changes in the tissue or organ's character. The changes may come from a defective blood supply or involve the deposition of calcium salts, fat, or fibrous material in the affected organ or tissue. Such a change in character and function of the particular part is considered a degenerative disease. As I have assured, some degenerative diseases caused by the lack of free blood flow through the vessels that are aided by the administration of chelation therapy will be discussed.

Diabetes is one of these disease reactions to poor circulation. It is the sixth most common cause of debilitation and death, contributing to 50 percent of all heart attacks and 25 percent of all strokes in the United States. Diabetics are prone to having their blood vessels clog with fat, and 98 percent of the victims suffer with diabetic complications, such as cataracts, heart disease, kidney damage, blindness, blood vessel damage, and nerve disorders. Most are overweight.

Patients with diabetes are treated with a course of chelation therapy by holistic physicians who follow a protocol devised by the American College of Advancement in Medicine in a manner that brings the patients back to eating more unprocessed foods. Certain foods are natural chelators such as bran, whole-grain wheat, oats, corn, cereals, lentils, beans, peas, peanuts, figs, dates, apples, and other rich sources of fiber and complex carbohydrates. The mineral chromium in the form of a glucose tolerance factor is another natural chelator for diabetics. Diabetics can also have their insulin requirements reduced by EDTA intravenous infusions.

In **gallstones**, a normally soluble component of bile separates and grows in the gallbladder, producing a predisposition to disease in 20 percent of the adult populations around the Western world. Women are affected four to one over men. Eighty-five percent of all gallstones are composed of cholesterol, whose concentration in the blood is reduced by chelation therapy. Besides lowering serum cholesterol, therefore, it also dissolves gallstones.

Kidney diseases related to circulation difficulties usually arise from narrowing of the renal artery, which is divided into smaller branches flowing through a kidney and its filtering units. One of the kidney pathologies, kidney stones, may be shrunk in size or made to disappear altogether by the kidney patient's employment of chelation therapy.

Chelating physicians have reported at recent semi-annual meetings of the ACAM that not only does chelation therapy not hurt the kidneys as had been reported in the past, but it actually aids in their improved function. Published in the *Journal of Holistic Medicine*, Volume 4, Number 2, Fall/Winter 1982, the article, "The Effect of EDTA Chelation Therapy Plus Supportive Multivitamin-Trace Mineral Supplementation Upon Renal Function: A Study of Serum Creatinine" by Drs. Edward W. McDonagh, Charles J. Rudolph, and Emanuel Cheraskin, specifies that of 383 people treated by these physicians with EDTA intravenous injections, no patient had any kidney damage, including those who began with impaired kidneys. In the article they state: "Hence, it would appear, within the limits of this study, that this therapeutic regimen [chelation therapy] is not nephrotoxic [damaging to the kidneys]. There is even a suggestion that this treatment procedure may improve kidney function." In Chapter Six on safety and side effects of chelation therapy, I will discuss more on the precautions to be taken for kidney patients.

Clots in the blood vessels can bring about strokes, phlebitis, pulmonary embolism, or varicose veins. Certain antioxidant nutrients, which I mentioned in the last chapter, also happen to be chelating agents. They are vitamin C, vitamin E, and selenium. Oral chelators such as these nutrients are often recommended by chelating doctors for patients who have blood clots. People experiencing trouble with the blood-clot problem called thrombophlebitis will probably have heparin added to the EDTA solution during their course of intravenous chelation treatment.

The **emphysemic patient** possesses microscopic air sacs of the lungs that have lost their elasticity. Air flows into them but cannot flow out as easily because of the narrowed diameter of the sac passageway. Because of this air entrapment, the victim tends to retain too much stale air. Like small balloons, tiny air bubbles take up space in the air sacs so that their thin walls become over-stretched to the point of rupture. Gas exchange is decreased. Emphysema leads to shortness of breath, overworking of the heart, and possible death. In addition to taking chelation therapy, which is an aid to blood transport, restoration of good nutrition is mandatory for this lung condition.

Cataracts are solidified forms of a person's normally transparent lenses, an opacity which acts like a curtain to prevent light rays from reaching the retina, the eye nerve, and the brain. Hardening of the arteries causes a partial blockage of the blood supply going to the eyes, and is frequently responsible for the cataracts. Cholesterol deposits are sometimes another cause. Chelation therapy is a specific adjunctive way to bring about a biochemical change for improvement of the eyes without resorting to cataract surgery.

Senility may involve atrophy of brain cells from cholesterol-filled plaques narrowing the brain blood vessels. Another manifestation of senility is Alzheimer's disease, a relentlessly progressive form of senile dementia now diagnosed in 5 to 10 percent of all people over sixty-five. Brain aluminum concentrations are four times higher than normal in patients with Alzheimer's disease, causing structural damage of nerve plaques and tangles. Tangles are clumps of filaments that form within the nerve cell body. Plaques are hard knots of debris marking the site of a burned-out nerve cell ending.

Chelation therapy is the only treatment available to restore a person to society once he or she gets **Alzheimer's disease**. Two kinds of chelating agents are used for the intravenous injection. Beside EDTA, which is readily given in the trained chelating doctor's office and requires no hospitalization, another chelator used is desferrioxamine. Donald R.C. McLachlan, M.D., professor of physiology and medicine at the University of Toronto, gives desferrioxamine infusions to Alzheimer's disease patients, twice daily. However, any of the chelating physicians listed in this book's appendix are qualified to attempt the reversal of Alzheimer's disease using the vastly tested, quite effective, and exceedingly safe EDTA. Desferrioxamine is rather untried to date.

In the arteriosclerotic disease, **macular degeneration**, blood is prevented from reaching the central part of the retina through the choroid capillaries. A blind spot results in the part of the vision that is used for looking directly at an object. Then the victim can no longer read, see the colors of objects, or recognize other people. Chelation therapy appears to bring back the circulation to such affected vision and improves it better than any other therapy now available—better than even eye surgery.

Varicose veins in the legs possess damaged valves that are supposed to lift the blood against gravity, prevent backflow, and return it to the heart. The cause of their damage could be bacterial infection, obesity, injuries that produce blood flow obstruction, poorly oxygenated venous blood, or metabolic waste products in the blood stream. Most of these may be overcome by enhancing vein circulation through increasing the blood nutrition to the veins themselves. You are able to accomplish this with either intravenous or oral chelation treatment.

Parkinson's disease, a slow, progressive condition of the basal ganglia located in the small center at the base of the brain, does not affect the major portion of the brain, so that the patient remains intelligent, is not paralyzed, and does not lose the ability to speak. Instead, he has tremors, stiffness, shuffling gait, and slowness of movement. Arteriosclerotic parkinsonism is just one of three types of the disease and occurs in the elderly. It responds fairly well to chelation therapy, especially in the disease's beginning stages. The pill-rolling effect in a newly diagnosed patient's fingers stops when the intravenous treatment is given.

Osteoporosis, the pronounced porousness of bones, more frequently happens in menopausal women. It is the cause of sudden bone fractures for no apparent reason. But bone recalcification can be stimulated by continued osteoblastic activity, which takes calcium from blood serum as a result of EDTA intravenous administration. Osteoblasts are the body's bone-forming cells.

With osteoblastic activity, soft tissue pathologic calcium in plaques continues to diminish in order to meet the need caused by this increased bone uptake of calcium. The renewed osteoblastic reaction produced after a series of chelation treatments can go on for up to three months. Serum calcium is continuously leached back into bones by activated osteoblasts with the result that the serum calcium has to be replenished by other body stores. It accomplishes this restoration by removing some of the calcium from soft tissue and pathological stores, such as calcium from arteries and around joints. Hardened arteries soften and widen. Arthritic joints get more mobile and stop hurting.

A therapeutic cycle in osteoporotic bone continues: (1) EDTA takes up serum calcium and disposes of it as waste, (2) the parathyroid hormone, parathormone, activates bone-forming cells, (3) bones grow stronger, (4) bones require more calcium for their build-up, (5) more atherosclerotic plaques give off loosely bound metastatic calcium to satisfy the osteoblasts' demand, (6) arteries soften, grow more flexible, and widen steadily in the process, and (7) the bone formation continues at an increased rate all the while keeping up the dissolution of metastatic calcium gathered from around the circulatory system.

Moreover, the bones and teeth get stronger, because ionic and metastatic calcium that may have avoided being grasped by the chelation claw go into reinforcing existing bone. Osteoporosis reverses.

Paget's disease is a chronic process of bone destruction, overgrowth, and new bone formation which occurs in the elderly and most frequently affects the skull, backbone, pelvis, and long bones. Frequently, hardening of the arteries and impaired blood supply to the bone exists. Chelation therapy works to relieve the pain and deformity associated with Paget's disease.

Hypertension is a symptom rather than a disease; it's an elevation of blood pressure far exceeding the normal body limits. Usually hypertension is present when the systolic pressure is above 140 and the diastolic exceeds 90. One of the quickest benefits you will witness from taking chelation treatment is a lowering of high blood pressure to normal.

PHYSIOLOGICAL CHANGES
FROM CHELATION THERAPY

A few patients of Antonia E.J. Monti, M.D., medical director of the El Cajon Medical Center, El Cajon, California, were victims of some of the degenerative diseases aided by chelation therapy. They experienced positive physiological changes from the treatment. For example, Alice Bradshaw of Jamul, California, had high blood pressure. She said, "After being treated with many drugs that either made me ill or were not effective, my diastolic blood pressure was as high as 130. After eight chelation treatments it has dropped as low as 80 [which is normal]."

Mr. R. R. Allen of El Cajon said, "My chest pain is gone and I feel a lot better after taking the chelation therapy. I have no pain or shortness of breath anymore. My eyesight is also much improved."

Herb R. Carlson of Rancho Mirage, California, now age 74, wrote: "Since I was about 24 years old, I have been under the care of internists and heart specialists in various areas of America. My work in sales management required intense action and resulting high stress. I had high blood pressure, heart angina, and finally two heart attacks 20 years ago. I also developed a bleeding ulcer nine years ago and was hospitalized. Four years ago I suffered four [successive] strokes which were absolutely devastating to me.

"All during these years," Mr. Carlson continued, "I was under the constant care of qualified physicians who used the same type of medications and treatments over and over again. Yet I became progressively worse. Then I was faced with heart surgery, also four years ago. At no time was I ever encouraged to do something on my own to lower my blood pressure. No one told me that something like chelation therapy could effectively control my angina and atherosclerosis.

"The only thing recommended was a life-threatening operation to provide better circulation to my heart and stop the angina. Here I was age 70 and told—the common remark from all those doctors— 'so what do you expect at this stage of life?'

"But then I studied the literature and talked to people who had undergone chelation therapy," said Mr. Carlson. "It appeared to me that this was the one treatment making common sense, a form of chemical Roto Rooter™ to clean out my arteries."

"Today, thanks to chelation therapy, at the advanced age of 74 years, I enjoy a vigorous life, more activity, better health, and work every day traveling in sales around Southern California. This chelation treatment has put new life in me and I heartily recommend that anyone who has heart problems seriously study the sort of book you're reading now. You can gain accurate knowledge from it. Then use the common sense and wisdom we are all endowed with to make the right decision to also enjoy [a] longer and more robust life and good health," Carlson continued.

"It takes courage to fly in the face of the opponents of chelation therapy at the American Medical Association. I did and am very happy for it."

Reverend Al Connell, the chaplain at El Cajon Valley Hospital, said, "In September 1978, I had four different cardiologists diagnose angina pectoris with 80 percent blockage of my coronary arteries. All four recommended potential bypass considerations. One of the cardiologists told me about chelation therapy and, even though he had taken the treatment for his own angina, could not openly recommend it. I then proceeded to have chelation treatment anyway, under my own advisement. This approach produced relief after only six treatments. By relief I refer to no more chest pains. This allowed me to cut my medications down 75 percent and ultimately 100 percent. After thirty-five treatments [by July 1, 1983], I am able to perform 85 percent of my normal work without pain."

Why is it that these patients of Dr. Monti's had such good results despite their initial conditions relating to hardening of the arteries? Because the treatment provides the body with a number of advantageous physiological effects. For instance, the treatment prevents the deposit of cholesterol in the liver, enhances sugar metabolism, and improves fat metabolism. It increases the excretion of cadmium from kidney cells, eliminates vascular spasm, and elevates serum magnesium by the mineral's better utilization from food sources. Moreover, intravenously administered EDTA alters the turnover rate of mucopolysaccharides for better function, helps to gather protein-connective tissue components, increases red blood cell membrane flexibility, prevents the fold-over effect in sickle cell anemia, and stops the anemia-producing red blood cell **rouleaux** formation. Rouleaux is red blood cell aggregation that cuts down on the amount of surface area provided for oxygen to occupy the cell.

Then, chelation therapy with EDTA augments the synthesis of collagen tissues, reduces the effects of rheumatoid arthritis pathology, improves capillary bed perfusion, thins basement cell membrane thickening for the diabetic's advantage, lowers blood viscosity, and lowers serum fats so that there is less chance of forming atherosclerotic plaque.

Not the least of its overcoming disease conditions includes the treatment's ability to cut down on the cross-linking of elastin, the major connective tissue protein of elastic structures such as tendons and skin. Since cross-linking of the body's macromolecules by free radicals and calcium is now known to be a basic aging mechanism, the individual who gets rid of cross linkers will see positive signs in his skin. Wrinkles tend to go away. (See Figures 4.1 and 4.2.)

Other internal functions that are improved by chelating the body systems include zinc metabolism, which is accomplished by raising the levels of usable unstable zinc in the food supply. It does this by improving the lactate dehydrogenase enzyme and nicotinamide adenine dinucleotide enzyme, both involved in degrading lactate and changing glycogen into glucose. Insulin requirements get reduced, too.

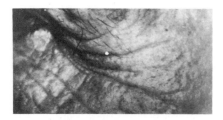
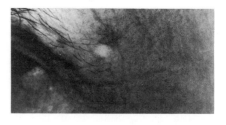

1. The corner of a patient's eye, depicting crow's-feet. The crow's-feet furrows were deeply wrinkled at the time of photographing, before being given chelation therapy by Dr. Charles Farr, medical director of the Genesis Medical Center of Oklahoma City, Oklahoma on August 12, 1974.

2. The same crow's-feet furrows, remarkably improved in appearance after chelation therapy, October 8, 1975. The skin appears smoother, younger, healthier, and has lost some of its wrinkles. This finding, which occurs in some people very rapidly and in others a little slower, is quite consistent.

Figure 4.1.   Crow's-feet, before and after chelation therapy.

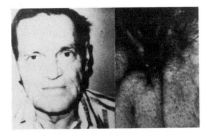
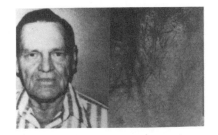

1. Dr. Charles Farr has photographed the "on-face" view of Mr. H.W. and a close-up view of the corner of the man's left eye area before he received chelation therapy, May 2, 1974.

2. Next, the same view taken August 3, 1974, after Mr. H.W. underwent a series of EDTA chelations shows him with less and shallower skin furrows, especially at the corner of the left eye.

Figure 4.2.   Skin, before and after chelation therapy.

The physiological effects of EDTA chelation therapy, or of almost any other chelator removing abnormal calcium deposits, do a variety of good things for the recipient's body. Blood cholesterol is lowered in the amount of 10 to 20 percent. There is an increase in the high-density lipoprotein (HDL) fraction or "good" blood cholesterol that results in an improved cholesterol/HDL ratio which measures your non-tendency to develop hardening of the arteries. The treatment reduces any irregularity in the heartbeat. It overcomes digitalis intoxication that may have accidentally been induced by your doctor. As I will point out in the chapter to follow, the studies of H. Richard Casdorph, M.D., Ph.D. of Long Beach, California, indicate that EDTA administered intravenously significantly improves the left ventricular ejection fraction, which is a measure of output of the heart. And there is a reversal of heart ST segment depression, which is a benefit for cardiac patients, independent of the amount of exercise they receive. The improvement in the circulation to the head and neck using IV and oral chelation treatment has also been demonstrated by the use of a non-invasive diagnostic technique known as oculoplethysmography.

All of the positive effects of EDTA infusions and other forms of chelation treatment have been documented in nearly 2,000 published medical journal and scientific articles. There is only one negative article on the subject, written by Drs. J. R. Kitchell, F. Palmon,

Jr., N. Aytan, and L. E. Meltzer and published in the *American Journal of Cardiology,* in 1963, under the title, "The Treatment of Coronary Artery Disease With Disodium EDTA. A Reappraisal." This single anti-chelation therapy article is cited over and over again by the treatment's enemies. It's the only printed rebuttal item they have to carry their arguments. Other than this piece, anything more that they have to say about chelation therapy administration usually is groundless rumor or false innuendo. In Chapter Eight on the chelation therapy mistake of organized medicine, I explain in detail how this 1963 clinical journal article is largely responsible for the absolute error in judgment displayed by American medicine in considering chelation treatment for atherosclerosis unacceptable. Establishment physicians are wrong simply because they are basing their judgments mostly on this one published article.

Anyone truly informed about chelation therapy must conclude that the criticism of it is mere nonsense babble, inasmuch as the various opponents don't have personal knowledge of the facts. Why may such a broad statement be made? Because opponents more often than not have never given the treatment to patients for eliminating hardening of the arteries, nor have they taken it for themselves as practically all chelating physicians have done to insure their own life extensions.

In the book, *Chelation Can Cure,* (Platinum Pen Publishers, 1983, paperback) by Edward W. McDonagh, D.O., the author states: "Those who would have you believe chelation is dangerous or ineffective should be totally ignored, UNLESS THEY HAVE HAD PERSONAL [emphasis Dr. McDonagh's] experience in administering this form of medical treatment. If they have never treated a patient with EDTA, or even seen a patient before and after chelation therapy, their advice is HEARSAY. Any lawyer or judge in this country can tell you quickly how much hearsay statements are worth."

CHAPTER FIVE
The Clinical Studies of Chelation Therapy

Rosie Matelan of Linesville, Pennsylvania, had developed a chronic infection at one side of the nail of her third finger, right hand, for which she sought medical treatment three separate times from different orthopedic surgeons. Each orthopedist, in turn, diagnosed that Mrs. Matelan was suffering from the degenerative disease known as lupus erythematosus (LE), which, lucky for her, was affecting the woman only in its mildest form.

Lupus erythematosus is a chronic inflammatory disease of connective tissue, involving the skin and various internal organs. Typically, there is a red scaly rash on the face, encompassing the nose and cheeks; arthritis; and progressive damage to the kidneys. Often the heart, lungs, and brain are also affected by progressive attacks of inflammation followed by the formation of scar tissue (fibrosis). In the mild form that Mrs. Matelan showed, her skin appeared to be the only organ affected. LE is regarded as an autoimmune disease (like AIDS) and can be diagnosed by the presence of abnormal antibodies in the blood stream, most easily detected by a test that reveals characteristic white blood cells (LE cells). While the disease is most often treated with corticosteroids, chelation therapy does a much better job but, unfortunately, orthodox medical practitioners invariably overlook this more effective mode of treatment. Moreover, corticosteroids complicate the situation with a large number of serious side effects, and chelation therapy has very few of a serious nature. (See Chapter Six.) In the case of lupus erythematosus, the same victims of mainstream medicine's neglect remain the ongoing victims of this degenerative disease.

When the third finger infection became especially troublesome for Rosie Matelan, in May 1982, the orthopedic surgeon she was visiting at the time extracted pus from it. Her whole right hand then began to swell and pain miserably. In July the finger turned black from gangrene well past the nail root area and eventually needed to be amputated. Around October 10, 1982, the woman's second and fourth fingers on her right hand also became infected at the nail edges. They too gradually began turning black. Matelan delayed a month and then sought help from Donald J. Mantell, M.D., who is in general and family practice in Evans City, Pennsylvania. Dr. Mantell performed a physical examination of the patient in his office on November 10, 1982, and found that her fourth finger was completely black with dry gangrene from the tip forward. The patient's second finger was slightly black, as well. And the doctor saw that her right hand's third finger had been cut off at the distal interphalangeal joint.

Dr. Mantell chose chelation therapy to treat this case of lupus erythematosus. Matelan received five chelation treatments at the doctor's office. "After the second chelation treatment," this chelating physician wrote to me in a letter, "her fingers were already much improved. The finger tips were less black and starting to drain. The fourth finger, which had been completely black, was developing pink granulation tissue at the proximal edge of the gangrenous border. Ordinarily I would not have believed the results if I had not seen them."

After taking those first five chelation treatments with Dr. Mantell, Matelan continued her therapy with another chelating physician who happened to be located closer to her home. James Lapcevic, D.O., Ph.D. of Grove City, Pennsylvania, provided the patient with thirty more chelation treatments.

To learn how the patient was progressing with lupus erythematosus of the skin, I contacted Dr. Mantell on September 15, 1983. He had kept in touch with this striking case and reported to me that the woman's fingers are cleared of the condition entirely with no trace of black gangrenous tissue present. All signs of her condition of lupus erythematosus of the skin are gone altogether. Any of the former dead skin and damaged underlying connective tissue has been replaced by pink new growth. She has full use of her nine remaining fingers. Today Mrs. Matelan is exceedingly happy over the turn of events as a result of having taken chelation therapy. The woman gave the chelating doctors and me approval to reveal her case history.

THE DEMAND FOR DOUBLE-BLIND STUDIES

The type of story you have just read, along with the other case histories in this book, are considered "anecdotal evidence" by establishment doctors. Those conservative physicians strictly following the traditional scientific method, as it is recognized in the United States, assign anecdotal evidence—even a patient report like Rosie Matelan's, which is supplied by two of their fellow medical doctors—no serious attention.

A major argument used by the anti-chelation forces is that physicians extolling chelation therapy have not carried out double-blind studies for the treatment. Alfred Soffer, M.D., former executive director of the American College of Chest Surgeons and a chief antagonist of chelation therapy, declares that there are no physician-authored articles on the treatment that he knows of, published in the last 100 years, with a controlled double-blind randomized prospectus trial reported in a reputable clinical journal. He also denies that any laboratory research on EDTA chelation administered IV has been valid. Dr. Soffer prefers that chelation therapy be tested in an investigational environment. But this earlier champion of the treatment, having in 1964 written the medical text *Chelation Therapy*, extolling its benefits for cardiovascular disease, but now with his back turned on the procedure, refuses to call for a clinical trial because he says that he knows of no new evidence of its effectiveness since he finished with his 1964 work. Perhaps letting his ego blind him to reality or just exhibiting pigheaded shortsightedness, Dr. Soffer is failing to recognize numbers of clinical studies on chelation therapy accomplished in the last twenty-five years and some already reported in the medical literature. You will know about a few of these studies by the time you finish reading this chapter. I have reported on one such study in Chapter Four showing that healthy kidneys are not harmed by chelation therapy and that impaired kidneys actually show functional improvement by EDTA infusion.

Along with chelation therapy foes like Dr. Soffer, the U.S. Food and Drug Administration (FDA) wants double-blind studies, as well. This agency's impatience with the doctors who are chelation therapy proponents is exhibited by its continuous harassment of those giving the treatment for atherosclerosis.

The FDA has a policy of demanding double-blind studies, even though they are impossible to carry out. FDA personnel state that those wanting approval for unproven remedies always say it is difficult to complete controlled double-blind trials. When asked about the hundreds of thousands of Americans and Canadians who have been successfully administered chelation therapy and shown greatly increased health improvement, the FDA says, "That's anecdotal evidence."

Dr. Soffer says, "Anecdotal evidence is bullshit!"

The attitude of these two anti-chelation exponents, supposedly representing expertise in medicine, is strange when you consider the excellent results experienced by patients with all kinds of degenerative diseases who have taken chelation therapy. They have little or no corresponding harmful side effects, either, something you will learn more about in Chapter Six.

It's also strange to consider that coronary artery bypass surgery has never been required by these same chelation therapy oppositionists to go through any double-blind studies. No one seems to talk about the statistical realities of bypass surgical dangers. An average range of every twenty-fifth to fiftieth person who accepts the bypass operation dies on the operating table. Over one-fourth of those having their chests split open experience terribly crippling complications for many months afterward. Within two years, 40 percent of the arterial bypass grafts close up so that the life-endangering operation possibly has to be done again, if the patient can take it. So, don't you wonder why there is a double standard that demands double-blind studies for chelation therapy and not for open heart surgery?

One of the reasons you cannot have double-blind controlled studies to test the efficacy of intravenous EDTA is that people not getting the real treatment would know it. There are certain minor reactions or telltale signs with IV chelation therapy. For example, you feel the need to urinate a lot while receiving the IV drip as your arteries clear of calcium and get rid of it through your urinary tract. Or, you might feel a tingling of the skin as the EDTA solution runs through your blood vessels. I will discuss other inconsequential side effects, as I mentioned before, in the next chapter.

Double-blind controlled studies on humans are not available now, either, simply because of a lack of financing for such investigations. No institutions have backed any double-blind tests for chelation treatment—not the federal government, medical schools, hospitals, universities, philanthropic organizations, foundations, pharmaceutical companies, or any other group—with cash grant allocations or research facilities. There is no interest in the institutions to perform such studies. They seemingly are uninformed about chelation therapy or, as with the pharmaceutical industry, this treatment competes too well against products or services bringing the institutions income.

Here is an illustration of the health institutions' ignorance of chelation therapy that took place September 7, 1983. Cheryl Hirsh, an editor at *Your Good Health* (Keats Publishing, New Canaan, Connecticut), was preparing an article on chelation treatment for the magazine's November or December 1983 issue. She knew of many proponents quite willing to testify in favor of the treatment and had included their remarks. Wanting to provide the reader with a balanced piece, however, the editor went looking for statements from some chelation therapy opponents. Cheryl could not find any. Her lack of treatment foes did not arise because of an insufficient number of physicians willing to spout the erroneous party line of organized medicine. No! Plenty of those hacks exist. In calling around to the big medical institutions, editor Hirsch learned that almost none of those working in traditionally practiced medicine even knows what chelation therapy is, what it does, how it's administered, or what it consists of. For example, a prominent doctor at Yale University School of Medicine answered, "Chelation therapy? I never heard of it!"

The irony of this situation is that Cheryl Hirsh telephoned me to put her onto a few enemies of chelation therapy. Having appeared in many lecture, radio, television, and print media debates with cardiologists, endocrinologists, and internists hostile to the treatment, I was able to assist this editor with sources for slandering a procedure that I know saves limbs and extends life. I did it in the cause of fairness to the uninformed other side.

CHELATED PATIENTS ARE THEIR OWN CONTROLS

If studies are to be performed, usually costing multi-millions of dollars, the expenses would have to be underwritten by individual chelating doctors. Such a situation is grossly unfair. Doctors in private practice usually don't have the financial resources. And it's improbable that such privately financed double-blind studies will ever occur! So where is the money to come from for the medical supplies, the different solutions and nutrients, the professional care, plus the extensive time investments involved?

And who will be the control group of human guinea pigs for the studies demanded? Real patients undergoing chelation therapy pay hard currency for fulfilling their health needs; no ethical chelating doctor is going to inject them with distilled water for its placebo effect without telling people they aren't receiving their money's worth. Would you pay for something you may not be getting? Would you consent to being part of a double-blind program when your body requires the repair mechanisms offered by the real chelation treatment?

H. Richard Casdorph, M.D., Ph.D. of Long Beach, California, to whom I have alluded in Chapter Four, contends that double-blind studies are unnecessary, since each patient legitimately receiving chelation therapy serves as his own control. Dr. Casdorph demonstrated this with radioisotope studies before and after treatments.

Elmer M. Cranton, M.D., medical director of the Mount Rogers Clinic of Trout Dale, Virginia, past president of the American Holistic Medical Association, additionally affirms that patients are their own controls. The two chelation experts are correct, for it's obvious! A large group of people about to undergo chelation therapy will take a series of clinical function tests as beginning baselines to show how their systems are impaired. Then their individualized series of EDTA infusions are administered over the time the patients require them. Next, after they have received the appropriate amount of chelation therapy the majority of the patient's symptoms are likely to just disappear. Their body systems are again checked and compared against the baseline studies performed just before the chelation care had been given. Now the patients have been used as their own controls, and they have received the full complement of required treatment. The people have not been fooled with placebos. They have been administered true therapy. They have been their own controls. Isn't it sufficient that gangrene has gone for potential amputees, angina no longer strikes the cardiacs, continually cold limbs have warmed and stayed that way, vision has been restored for those with macular degeneration, insulin dosage has lowered or been eliminated for diabetics, the senile elderly again recognize their children, leg muscle cramps stop coming on for lovers of movement, and much more of a restorative nature makes its appearance for these patients who have taken chelation therapy?

Why is so-called anecdotal evidence so bad? Is the integrity of a reporting doctor in question? Don't the patients' reactions, feelings, symptoms, body signs, and laboratory readings count for anything? And if some kind of placebo effect is the source of their healing, well, what's wrong with that? Isn't it healing that we are after?

A major difference exists between traditionally practiced allopathic medicine and the more current holistic medicine. Allopathic medicine, which requires double-blind controlled studies, treats parts of a person like his liver or a broken bone; it also treats mostly classes of people such as babies or women; it concerns itself almost exclusively with disease and not with wellness. Holistic medicine, in contrast, cares for the whole individual, the entire sum of one's body parts; it is not involved with people classifications. It goes forward in health care to preventing problems before they arise. Double-blind controlled studies conducted among really sick patients anathematizes the concept of holism, and hardly could be accepted by a holistic thinker. In other words, double-blind controlled studies are nonholistic; trying for the placebo effect is dishonest.

Besides which, contrary to what enemies of the treatment have implied, benefits derived for the patient from his or her use of chelation therapy do not involve the placebo effect. This is proven by a veterinarian, Dr. L.S. McKibbin, practicing at the Wheatley Hall Farm Ltd. in Wheatley, Ontario, Canada. Dr. McKibbin is noted for getting race horses to run faster. He described to me how he uses his skill as a chelating veterinarian to increase the speed of thoroughbreds with intravenous injections of EDTA. Are the horses exhibiting a placebo effect? Do the horses know what substance is running through their blood vessels? When chelation nutrient substances are given to them in their hay, are they responding mentally in the form of faster running time? Horse manure!

ANOTHER CONTROLLED STUDY METHOD IS PROPOSED

In a December 1980 editorial published by the official voice of the California Medical Association (CMA), the *Western Journal of Medicine* in the article entitled "Scientific Methods in Medicine" acknowledges that the modern double-blind controlled studies have significant limitations. The CMA, an avowed enemy of chelation therapy, confesses that it is often impossible to control all the "linear process" in such double-blind studies. It often takes too much time to find a use for the study's conclusions in medical practice. The editorial writer discusses a second scientific method that is gaining widespread acceptance and may be better for investigating chelation therapy. The other method draws its conclusions from some practical epidemiological studies, such as how medicine relates the elevated incidence of lung cancer to the increase in smoking among certain populations.

In objectively studying the clinical effects of chelation therapy, the scientists would simply observe patients for years to find out if they die at an older age than non-chelated patients. Would they require less hospitalization or have fewer heart attacks, cancer, adult onset diabetes, and other degenerative diseases than those people not chelated? Meantime, the people who want chelation therapy would not be denied getting it by the standard devious practices, such as restricting their health insurance payments, limiting the medical practice rights of physicians who would render chelation therapy services, or saying nasty and untrue things about the treatment on the media as had Ted Turner's Cable News Network April 23, 24, 25, 26, 27, 1983. (I was interviewed at the Evers Health Center in Cottonwood, Alabama, by the CNN-TV hosts, who came in with treachery in their hearts smiling sweetly and acting friendly. They did a double-crossing hatchet job on Dr. Evers and the whole chelation therapy movement. They never broadcasted my interview, which praised the treatment.)

The editorial writer who composed the *Western Journal of Medicine* article I have referred to believes that medicine needs some method other than double-blind controlled studies for testing the efficacy of new remedies against disease. He says that the scientific method has to develop another model "because in health and illness, there are so many changing factors at work in any given moment." The editor anticipates that our rapidly developing computer technology will make possible the calculations needed for the new type of research. Out of high technology, another scientific method for medicine will be better applied to the ever-changing interactions of, as yet, poorly understood multifactual aspects of health and disease. For the chelation treatment of the cardiovascular sick, in particular, it is essential that this new method be developed quickly, even if not perfectly, so that it may produce timely results in terms of the life expectancy of so many patients.

THE FIRST CLINICAL STUDY BY AN ACAM PHYSICIAN

Although most doctors involved with organized medicine, the governmental agencies that use income tax dollars to support medical research, plus a variety of establishment institutions and foundations all talk about controlled double-blind studies as offering the only conclusive proof of the efficacy of chelation therapy, an increasing amount of laboratory experiments and private clinical investigations are currently throwing light on what the treatment can do for cardiovascular patients.

The laboratory work and efficacious treatments are being carried out with the use of highly sophisticated machines measuring the flow of blood before and after people receive chelation therapy. These are not double-blind or single-blind investigations. They are ordinary clinical observations recorded as changes occur in patients undergoing chelation therapy. The results are sent along for storage and eventual publication by the ACAM. These studies are being paid for out of the private practice time and income of individual chelating physicians who recognize the need for some type of controlled study mechanism. Without support from established institutions, they are attempting to fill some of the requirements of bonafide research.

One of the first physicians reporting on his research efforts to the spring 1979 scientific conference of the American College of Advancement in Medicine was psychiatrist Lloyd Grumbles, M.D., of Philadelphia. Dr. Grumbles employed the Baird System 77 Multicrystal Computerized Radioisotope Camera to measure and show through colored photographs the blood as it flowed through the brains or hearts of twenty patients. In these tests very short-lived radioisotopes were injected into the patients before and after they received chelation therapy for their infirmities.

The multicrystalline gamma isotope camera that Dr. Grumbles used took four pictures per second in a series of multiple photographs. Following just one second of photography, the individual patient's internal carotid arteries were outlined. In three more seconds the entire brain came into view, outlined in brilliant red and yellow colors. At five seconds an observer was able to visualize the individual's blood coming in and rushing out of his brain tissue.

Of the twenty people tested, over 80 percent of them had symptomatic relief of their heart or brain problems, including the near-total reversal of Alzheimer's disease. Being a psychiatrist, Dr. Grumbles was most keenly interested in the cerebral symptom improvements, but he also was amazed by the elimination of heart trouble in his chelated patients. He is able to show these improvements by verified measurements supplied by the Baird System 77 camera. I have seen his films. For example, one male patient, Elvis Powell of Camden, New Jersey, age 55, who had been referred to Dr. Grumbles by a neurosurgeon, had experienced repeated severe transient ischemic attacks that temporarily paralyzed him on one side of the body and made him unable to speak (called aphasia). Transient ischemic attack (TIA) is a temporary decrease in the supply of blood to a portion of the brain from arterial spasm or microemboli that have congregated in a local area, usually at a rough spot in the artery, so that blood flow is cut off, and symptoms develop. TIAs act selectively on various parts of the body because different parts of the brain control these body parts.

This TIA patient had been rushed to the hospital many times prior to finally being sent for treatment to Dr. Grumbles. In his first brain study, the man's brain was only faintly outlined after four seconds when ordinarily the colors should have been brilliant. At five seconds, when blood should have been rushing through his brain, Mr. Powell had blood merely leaking in. He was in imminent danger of having severe cerbrovascular disease symptoms, such as stroke, senile dementia, Alzheimer's disease, or mental illness.

The chelating psychiatrist chose the only treatment available to effect improvement of the patient's brain blood supply. After receiving twenty IV infusions of EDTA, the man submitted to another computerized radioisotope series of photographs. Now, his brain was nicely outlined in just three seconds and, looking at his photographs, you can see the arteries filling. After taking another twenty chelation treatments—forty in all—another test indicated that in four seconds, shown by the photograph's brilliant colors, normal blood flow had permanently returned to Powell's brain. Also, charged gamma particles that had measured only 297 before the start of chelation therapy, elevated to 1,666. (The particle count for a really healthy brain is about 2,768).

This man has required no more emergency trips to the hospital for help with TIAs from the end of his 1979 treatment to now. There is no doubt in the minds of the patient and his doctor that chelation therapy saved the man's life. Additionally, for ten years prior to chelation treatment, Powell had suffered with angina pectoris and emphysema. He usually had visited physicians for these two conditions about every six months. He did not need their attention any longer. For purposes of providing a finished report for this book, Elvis Powell went for a checkup of his former chest diseases. To their amazement, the same orthodox medical specialists who had treated him before he underwent chelation therapy expressed their astonishment that they could find absolutely no evidence of the pathology previously bringing on his angina and emphysema.

Incidentally, even though Elvis Powell, Mrs. Powell, and Dr. Lloyd Grumbles are firmly convinced that chelation therapy saved the man's life, he has been unable to get any health insurance policy reimbursement for his chelation therapy medical bills. The health insurance company says that it doesn't recognize chelation treatment as "usual and customary," and it refuses to pay for treatment rendered on a preventive basis. If he had sustained a stroke, the company assures this policy holder that it would have reimbursed Powell's medical care. Please take note that the man has "sickness" insurance and not so-called "health" insurance. Is this the type of coverage that you are buying?

Radioisotope studies with the multicrystal computerized camera
are probably even more reliable than the angiography used as a
standard in coronary artery bypass surgery. Reasons for this accu-
racy are that there is subjective doctor interpretation of the multicrystal photographs as with the angiologist interpreting an angiogram; plus, the computer reads out the blood flow by drawing a
graph that exactly shows how quickly the blood comes in and out of
the body part.

Dr. Grumbles is skilled sufficiently to read the results, but he
prefers to send them to the Spitz Clinic in Philadelphia, where they
are interpreted by a nuclear radiologist who has no particular interest in chelation therapy. That way, the readouts for these twenty
patients showing excellent health improvements have come from
an unbiased medical source. They are unquestionable! Unfortunately, many of the uninformed establishment doctors opposed to
chelation therapy are not familiar with the advanced diagnostic
techniques utilizing the Baird System 77 Multicrystal Computerized
Radioisotope Camera and don't seem to be interested in the Grumbles' studies.

ADDITIONAL CLINICAL STUDIES ARE PRESENTED

At nearly the same time Dr. Grumbles was performing his studies,
biotoxicologist Bruce W. Halstead, M.D., of Colton, California, was
starting similar before-and-after brain studies on thirteen chelated
patients in the neurosurgical department at Loma Linda University
School of Medicine. He documented his results at two separate
ACAM science conferences in 1980. Dr. Halstead's studies indicated
about an 82 percent improvement in the blood transit time, the
period it takes a gamma particle to get into the brain and out again.

Internist and cardiologist H. Richard Casdorph, M.D., Ph.D.,
who is Assistant Clinical Professor of Medicine at the University of
California Irvine School of Medicine and Chief of Medicine at Long
Beach Community Hospital and currently President of ACAM, had
practiced traditionally until he came upon the excellent health enhancement afforded by chelation therapy. Dr. Casdorph followed
the results from chelation treatment for four years before he decided
to incorporate it into his cardiovascular practice. To prove to himself
that the treatment wasn't producing improvements through any

placebo effect, he elected studies similar in method to those per-formed by Dr. Halstead and Dr. Grumbles.

On fifteen patients with well-documented impairment of cerebral blood flow, Dr. Casdorph utilized the isotope technetium 99m with the scintillation camera manufactured by Searle Radiographics. His studies were carried out on patients who had obstruction of brain blood circulation resulting in some definite brain disorder, such as dementia, senility, or other mind problems. Employing the radio-isotopes I have mentioned, the internist studied individuals' brains before and after chelation therapy and in every case confirmed the results of Dr. Grumbles. "All 15 patients improved clinically, includ-ing those with little or no improvement in [measured] cerebral blood flow," he wrote in his paper that was published in the *Journal of Holistic Medicine*, Volume 3, Number 2, Fall/Winter 1981.

The one patient who failed to show measured blood flow increase had been the repeated victim of transient ischemic attacks (TIAs) prior to chelation therapy. The TIAs disappeared entirely during and after treatment, wrote Dr. Casdorph.

Another of his patients was a "51-year-old white female with documented schizophrenia. She was hospitalized because of exac-erbation of back pain which subsequently proved to be due to chronic disc degeneration," the researcher said. The woman was incorporated into Dr. Casdorph's blood flow study and showed up as conspicuously abnormal in her thinking, actions, and cerebral vascular measurements. After she had received thirteen EDTA infu-sions, there was a marked improvement in the schizophrenic's brain blood flow. After twenty infusions had been delivered, the schizophrenia tended to go away. The patient's depression, her desire for isolation, the compulsion to sleep for long periods, intro-version, and other mind derangements all got better, too. She be-came more outgoing, cheerful, and for the first time was able to drive to the doctor's office by herself. Her family reaped the benefits of her newly found personality. And the woman expressed surprise that her slipped disc difficulty just stopped producing pain.

A third woman, at 72 years, had long-standing hypertension and computerized axial tomography (CAT) scan evidence of cerebral atrophy. CAT is a diagnostic radiology recording of "slices" of the brain anatomy that are integrated by computer to give a cross-sectional image. CAT scanning is without risk to the patient. This woman that Dr. Casdorph examined was confused and senile. She was experiencing delusions with hallucinations and often failed to recognize her husband to whom she had been married for over fifty years. When she walked out to the sidewalk in front of her home, she could not find her way back along the short path to her door. Sadly, the patient's husband was considering putting her in an institution for the brain-damaged elderly.

Chelation therapy saved this woman, who is plainly described in the published clinical journal paper, from succumbing to the living death of senility. After receiving only six IV injections with EDTA, Dr. Casdorph reports that her symptoms cleared. The patient became completely oriented and rational. It was no longer necessary to consider her for institutionalization. She also had improvement in her vision. Treatment continued and, much to the doctor's surprise, there was no significant increase in the patient's brain blood flow even with twenty infusions. However, when the treatment number reached twenty-six, suddenly the blood flowed well through her cerebral arteries.

The average number of chelation treatments for reversing senility and Alzheimer's disease seems to be in ranges between thirty and eighty, depending on the amount of nerve cell deterioration existing in the individual's brain. I report this treatment range to you from records kept among some 400 chelating physicians whom I have interviewed. They are steadily submitting clinical information in study groups sponsored by the ACAM.

With so much success recorded for cerebral disease, Dr. Casdorph decided to embark on a study of patients suffering from coronary artery disease. He performed research with eighteen patients having documented arteriosclerotic heart disease. The clinician writes, "A statistically significant improvement in the left ventricular ejection fraction occurred in essentially all of the patients to whom the drug [EDTA] was administered." An ejection fraction refers to the efficiency of the heart's left ventricle as a pump.

"The radioactive studies were performed in the nuclear medicine department of Long Beach Community Hospital," Dr. Casdorph said in his next clinical paper on chelation therapy. "In this study, each patient serves as his own control, being studied before and at the end of the prescribed course of chelation therapy . . . All patients improved clinically and in all but two there was a complete subsidence of chest pains . . . One patient who did not have complete relief of chest pains was [someone] who had had two previous open heart surgical procedures. Even so, during the course of chelation therapy her cardiac symptoms were markedly ameliorated."

CHELATING PHYSICIANS CAN'T GET
THEIR STUDIES PUBLISHED

The results of this second Casdorph study on heart problems and chelation therapy was also published in the *Journal of Holistic Medicine* following the quarterly issue presenting the brain study. But Dr. Casdorph had attempted first to get his two scientific papers published in the *New England Journal of Medicine* and then in the *Annals of Internal Medicine*. Both of these medical library indexed journals, which would have made current chelation therapy information available to establishment physicians, turned down the well-written material. Yet, in the past Dr. Casdorph has published letters or articles in both of those journals. The internal medicine journal is the official organ for the American College of Physicians of which Dr. Casdorph is not only a member but a fellow. He also attempted to present his paper to the American College of Chest Surgeons and was refused.

The situation meeting this highly qualified internist and cardiologist is typical of what befalls doctors wanting to report their results using chelation therapy to their colleagues. They cannot get published in standard, referenced, indexed medical journals. That is why, when your own doctor goes to his medical library to look up published information on chelation therapy in esteemed clinical journals, he or she won't find any with current dates of publication. All standard and commonly read journals stopped accepting articles on the benefits of chelation treatment in 1968. In Chapter Eight, I shall discuss why and how this happened.

"Dr. Casdorph has impeccable medical credentials. He conducted an excellent scientific study using the latest diagnostic techniques of radionucleide perfusion with technetium to evaluate cardiac function by determination of left ventricular ejection fraction, and he did this expensive study before and after a series of EDTA chelation treatments," wrote a fellow chelating physician, Warren M. Levin, M.D., who is medical director of the World Health Medical Group in New York City, in a letter of protest to the executive director of the American College of Physicians.

"His results on 16 out of 18 patients with arteriosclerotic heart disease are exciting and highly significant. The chances are less than five in 10,000 that these results could have occurred by chance. Because of the controversy surrounding chelation therapy, Dr. Casdorph expected to have difficulty getting this work published. What is worse, his fears were totally realized, and he has been unable to get even a summary letter published in any prestigious medical journal," Dr. Levin continued. "This, I think, is the best answer to the critics who say, 'if the therapy is so good, why don't you publish?' The fact that the full article was accepted for publication by the *American Journal of Holistic Medicine* is certainly no satisfaction since the physicians who read that journal are doctors who already believe in and use this controversial type of therapy, or are at least open to reading about it. Most importantly, however, this Journal [of the American Holistic Medical Association] is not indexed in the references to use in medical libraries for people who are attempting to do research in a subject."

Elmer Cranton, M.D., of Trout Dale, Virginia, who was editor of the *Journal of Advancement in Medicine*, said that the editorial staff of a main line medical journal will publish only those items that fit into their preconceived notions of how things should be. Such an indexed journal is not likely to expose the ordinary physician to an abundance of information to change the status quo. This has been the entire history of medicine, Dr. Cranton pointed out. Conservatism is the watchword for the editorial boards of organized medicine's magazines, journals, and its other periodicals.

"Chelation therapy does work," says Dr. Cranton. "It is safe. It is effective. And it is a persecuted treatment, much discriminated against by narrow-minded establishment doctors who don't want to hear about it. They can come up with all kinds of reasons why they should not recognize chelation therapy, but none of them are valid. Organized medicine is reactionary in terms of accepting new ideas unless [they are] something glamorous or revenue-producing such as coronary bypass operations or something else that results from personal research which enhances its vested interests."

THE NEWEST MEDICAL STUDIES ON CHELATION TREATMENT

The American College of Advancement in Medicine (ACAM) has on record somewhat more than 18,000 before-and-after thermographic evaluations of Americans with circulatory impairment involving peripheral vascular and/or cerebral vascular studies of individual patients. Thermographic evaluations involve the use of a registering thermometer called the **thermograph**, one form of which records every variation of temperature by means of a stylus, moving with the mercury in a tube, and registering the mercury's rise and fall on a circular temperature chart turned by clockwork. The picture produced by the thermograph is called a **thermogram**, providing a regional temperature map of the body or an organ. The thermogram is made without direct contact but is filmed by infrared sensing devices. If you are one of the Americans having had a non-invasive thermogram taken, it is measuring your radiant heat, and thus your recorded effective blood flow, when the room temperature has been kept constantly cool.

Then the ACAM has follow-up studies of these same thermographed patients long after the chelation treatment had been concluded. ACAM physicians have also furnished their College's archives with extensive studies of patients' plethysmograms, ultrasound Doppler analyses, and stress electrocardiograms. These studies indicate marked improvement in chelated patients' blood flow and are open for scrutiny to any institution, physician, and governmental agency willing to invest time in looking at them.

Even more than this research work, with the recent advent of the radioisotope blood flow scans, using technetium 99m and the Baird System 77 or other multicrystal computerized camera, the various studies by Drs. Grumbles, Halstead, and Casdorph and the additional studies I will describe in this section are available for duplicating. These objective data, as well as the clinical records furnished in the last twenty years by about 1,000 chelating physicians of hundreds of thousands of American patients, are enabling ACAM members to conclusively agree that EDTA chelation therapy is highly effective at increasing blood circulation in people suffering from impairment as a result of occlusive vascular disease.

The McDonagh, Rudolph, Cheraskin Studies

Published in the April 1982 issue of the *Journal of the International Academy of Preventive Medicine*, Volume VII, Number 1, pages 5-12, E.W. McDonagh, D.O.; C.J. Rudolph, Ph.D., D.O.; and E. Cheraskin, M.D., D.M.D., indicated in "The Effect of Intravenous Disodium Ethylene Diamine Tetraacetic Acid (EDTA) Upon Blood Cholesterol in a Private Practice Environment" that 142 of their patients treated with IV EDTA and supportive multivitamin-trace mineral supplementation had elevated blood cholesterol levels reduced on the average about 14 percent within two to four weeks. Those with the higher levels decreased about twice as much (17 percent) versus those with the lower initial values (9 percent).

Adding to the research studies, Drs. McDonagh, Rudolph, and Cheraskin published "An Oculocerebrovasculometric Analysis of the Improvement in Arterial Stenosis Following EDTA Chelation Therapy" in the Spring/Summer 1982 issue of the *Journal of Holistic Medicine*, Volume 4, Number 1, pages 21-23, in which they state: "Fifty-seven patients were evaluated objectively for cerebral vascular arterial occlusion before and after an average of 28 intravenous infusions of disodium ethylene diamine tetraacetic acid. Measurements of arterial occlusion were made with the relatively simple, noninvasive oculocerebrovasculometric analysis. Cerebrovascular arterial occlusion diminished by an average of 18 percent (from a mean of 28% to a mean of 10%) following therapy. Eighty-eight percent of patients treated with EDTA chelation therapy showed objective improvements in cerebrovascular blood flow."

These fifty-seven patients, thirty-four men ranging from 23 to 83 years old, and twenty-three women from 48 to 77 years old, were the victims of chronic degenerative disorders. Blood flow to their brains was measured with oculocerebrovasculometry (OCVM), a unique non-invasive tonometric system for detection of arterial insufficiency (stenosis). OCVM measures fluid pressures behind and within the eyeball to record the ophthalmic arterial pressure that, when compared to the brachial blood pressure, provides an accurate assessment of carotid artery occlusive disease, which could produce headaches or stroke, cerebrovascular occlusive disorders that might bring on senility, and ocular vascular pathology, which is responsible for some forms of blindness. The people in this study, all receiving chelation therapy, had their clogged arteries unblocked to the head and neck so that their brains once again received their full complement of blood.

Drs. McDonagh, Rudolph, and Cheraskin published "The Homeostatic Effect of EDTA With Supportive Multivitamin Trace Mineral Supplementation Upon High-Density Lipoproteins (HDL)" in *The Journal of the Osteopathic Physicians and Surgeons of California*, Volume 8, Number 2, Spring 1982 issue. In this study, 356 patients suffering with chronic degenerative problems were treated with IV EDTA plus a full nutritional and exercise program. The group, 178 males and 178 females, ranged in age from 14 to 84. Their high-density lipoproteins (HDL), the so-called "good" HDL, averaged before the study at 56 milligrams percent (mg %). The lower the HDL blood content, the higher is the cardiovascular risk. The HDL levels of this group of patients are shown in Table 5.1.

In all patients having low HDL scores, their blood HDL levels elevated an average range of 31 to 41 percent upon receiving a course of treatment with EDTA chelation therapy.

The Van der Schaar Studies

The internationally respected cardiovascular surgeon, P. J. van der Schaar, M.D., of Leyden, Holland presented his paper, "A Cardiovascular Surgeon Looks at Chelation Therapy," to the 1983 spring conference of the ACAM. Dr. van der Schaar has the unique position of practicing orthodox cardiovascular surgery both in his native Netherlands and at St. Luke's Hospital in Houston, Texas, with which he has been affiliated since 1976. In Holland, he utilizes

Table 5.1 Levels of High-Density Lipoproteins (HDL) in the Blood

HDL Level (mg percent)	Status	Number of Subjects
26	Dangerously at risk.	4 (1%)
26-35	High risk.	21 (6%)
36-44	Moderate risk.	58 (16%)
45-59	Average risk.	137 (39%)
60-74	Below average risk.	83 (23%)
75+	Protected for longevity.	53 (15%)

EDTA chelation therapy for the treatment of heart disease, peripheral vascular disease, and other blood vessel occlusions. He sees in this treatment a large part of the medical wave of the future. Dr. van der Schaar is a member of many professional medical organizations including the American Society of Thoracic Surgeons.

In late May 1983, Dr. van der Schaar reported to the ACAM physicians, "I started to administer chelation therapy to patients with inoperable peripheral vascular disease, in November 1981. My immediate results were encouraging and now the major part of my practice includes EDTA chelation therapy. I have already given more than 4,000 infusions and have produced a study of the first 111 consecutive patients. My report here is on the impressive results that I have witnessed. The people were divided into four categories: fifty with predominantly atherosclerotic peripheral vascular disease [blockage to blood circulation in the limbs], forty with predominantly atherosclerotic coronary artery disease, ten with cerebral vascular disease, and eleven with various other circulatory diseases. The minimum number of infusions was twenty and the maximum was fifty," he said.

"I had angiograms or Doppler studies available to me in most cases; furthermore, the peripheral vascular disease patients were classified into four classes to make judgments about their improvements with receiving chelation therapy," Dr. van der Schaar continued. "Those with the most severe intermittent claudication exhibited the best progress. My parameters indicate an average physical improvement of five times against symptoms for these chelated patients. Any that did not improve had refused to refrain from smoking, failed to keep the prescribed diet, and didn't take their usual oral chelating food supplements [prescribed when a physician follows the protocol of ACAM, which Dr. van der Schaar does].

"The forty coronary artery disease patients underwent coronary angiography and stress testing. The largest group of improvements occurred for those who suffered greatly with angina pectoris. The category of ten with cerebral vascular disease had been suffering from TIA, loss of memory, stroke, headache, hypertension, bad vision, and dizziness. To be considered improved, three signs of symptoms had to disappear." Dr. van der Schaar showed with slides that most of these patients eliminated at least three symptoms, and he considered them improved.

The last group of patients in the van der Schaar study had been victimized by a variety of circulatory-associated disorders, such as multiple sclerosis or parkinsonism, and they also experienced subjective improvements. "The patient with multiple sclerosis felt stronger and did not experience any deterioration in the last ten months, which he considers a definite improvement over the preceding years," the cardiovascular surgeon said. "The patients with Raynaud's disease showed a definite improvement in peripheral [blood] perfusion when chelation therapy is continued at intervals of three to four weeks."

Referring to people who require surgical intervention to save their lives or limbs, Dr. van der Schaar points out, "Where an operation is not possible, the best results are invariably obtained with first using chelation therapy. For example, in five of my patients the surgeon had already decided to amputate their limbs and in only one patient this actually needed to take place [after they had received chelation therapy].

The Sehnert, Clague Studies

In August 1983, Ann F. Clague, Ph.D., a therapeutic nutritionist and executive director of the Health & Wellness Center of Bloomington, Minnesota, and Keith W. Sehnert, M.D., the center's medical consultant and author of several books including *How To Be Your Own Doctor . . . Sometimes* (Grosset and Dunlap, New York, 1975), completed a study of chelated patients that was designed to gather data consistent with testing recommendations proposed for physicians who belong to ACAM. Drs. Clague and Sehnert studied a total of 216 patients, ranging in age from twenty-four to eighty-four, 159 men and 57 women, targeted with a variety of occlusive vascular disorders. They suffered from coronary heart disease, arteriosclerosis, peripheral vascular disease, hypertension, and cerebrovascular disease.

These cardiovascular-impaired patients received chelation therapy after undergoing diagnostic testing to establish a baseline for their health problems. Of the 216, 141 received ten IV injections with EDTA, 87 took twenty chelation treatments, 30 had thirty treatments, and 5 received forty. Treatments consisted of the doctors providing three grams (gm) of EDTA plus multivitamin-trace elements in a twice-weekly intravenous infusion that lasted for four hours, each time. The average number of treatments given was twenty-five, and daily oral vitamin-mineral supplements were prescribed. The supplements were continued at home by the individual patient for 90 to 160 days and were accompanied by a high bulk, nutritionally balanced diet.

Drs. Sehnert and Clague report that chest pains from angina pectoris and leg pains from intermittent claudication were markedly reduced for the chelated patients when these pains were compared before and after chelation therapy. The clinicians state the following: "The classic symptoms of occlusive vascular disease abated or disappeared in the majority of the patients in our study by the time they had received 20 to 30 treatments. The typical patient prior to chelation therapy had angina in two blocks, but after receiving 40 treatments could walk two miles without inducing chest or arm pain or distress."

The clinicians also point out that the type and number of drugs a person is forced to take is an effective indicator of how sick he or she is. "In assessing the improvement of any patient with cardiovascular disease (particularly those with life-threatening and frightening conditions such as coronary arteriosclerosis, hypertension and peripheral occlusive disease), the number of medications needed each day for relief of symptoms is a useful clinical indicator. Patients in this study were able to substantially reduce their needs for nitroglycerine and other medications. The 'other medication' category included nitrates, beta blockers, calcium antagonists, and antihypertensives," they wrote in their unpublished paper. (I possess an original copy, supplied for my review and comments, and presented here with the researchers' permission.) The excellent paper has been submitted for publication by clinical journals that have a prestigious board of medical editors as referees and are commonly read by the American medical profession. We hope that the Sehnert, Clague scientific paper will find a placement for the enlightenment of physicians in your community so as to break through the existing wall of prejudice against this life-sustaining treatment with injectable and oral chelating agents.

During the Sehnert and Clague studies, at intervals of ten chelation treatments, twenty treatments, and so on, each patient was directed to refrain from taking any oral calcium supplements on the day of a urine test. During this time the individual collected his or her urine for twenty-four hours. The specimen was sent to a clinical laboratory for analysis. The overall results for these patients showed a gradual increase in a dumping of calcium into the urine and out of the body that reached a peak at the twentieth treatment for the men and the thirtieth treatment for the women. Then this calcium dumping subsided after the chelation's initial artery-cleansing effect.

Additional beneficial evidence of patient improvement recorded by Drs. Sehnert and Clague was the drop in elevated blood pressure for any patients troubled with hypertension. They wrote, "The results of our study showed [blood pressure] decreases in both arms and the segmental (thigh, knee, ankle) pressures of both legs. An average decrease of 11.3 mm/Hg [millimeters of mercury] and 2.1 mm/Hg were found in male and female systolic arm pressures . . . The difference in the segmental pressures was even greater, dropping from a mean of 178.33 to 141.5 (26.8 mm/Hg) in the men." Thus, this study affirms that chelation therapy is effective in restoring high blood pressure back to normal and keeping it there.

In conclusion, the investigating clinicians say in their paper: "This study offers a preliminary report about a group of patients undergoing chelation with EDTA . . . The conclusion to be drawn is that in the dosage of 3 gm EDTA per day chelation is a safe and effective modality for occlusive vascular disorders. This therapy appears to enhance renal [kidney] blood flow, increase the output of urinary calcium, and lower the blood pressure in the arms and legs. It substantially lessens the requirements for nitroglycerin and other cardiovascular medications used for relief of angina. Patients in the program reported marked improvement in daily exercise tolerance."

A TEXAN WHO KNOWS CHELATION THERAPY HAS VALUE

Earl Lathrop of Amarillo, Texas, is a 53-year-old truck driver. In 1980 it was necessary for Mr. Lathrop to quit driving because he was experiencing chest pain that ended with consecutive heart attacks striking him in 1980 and 1981. He suffered from high blood pressure, too.

Hospitalization was forced on the man because of several more coronary artery problems, such as swelling, shortness of breath, and a total inability to do anything of a strenuous nature. His doctors therefore recommended that Lathrop undergo open heart surgery. Knowing of the high mortality rate of coronary artery by-pass recipients, this was one risk the big Texan did not want to take. He had heard too many horror stories about complications after heart surgery or death occurring during the operation.

The cardiac patient had been swallowing a lot of different drugs that he thought might help him. They had been prescribed as the only thing available short of having his breast bone split apart for the operation. He found, however, that these various drugs were causing many uncomfortable side effects. There was no way, for instance, that Lathrop could walk even a small distance from room to room in his house without feeling extremely short of breath or feeling angina pain.

One day luck turned his way when the patient heard of chelation therapy. His family members brought him the information, and he agreed that he was willing to try anything before having to settle on chest surgery. Lathrop then recalled the stories about this "detergent treatment for the arteries" and how it had done some good for other people in his same condition.

Lathrop sought out the services of two chelating physicians who work together at the Doctors Clinic in Amarillo, Texas, Gerald M. Parker, D.O., and John T. Taylor, D.O. Dr. Parker became his physician in September 1982. The patient was given an extensive physical examination including laboratory testing, non-invasive clinical testing, and a complete circulatory workup using the latest diagnostic equipment. A baseline series of test readings of his body systems was arrived at for comparison use in the future. Dr. Parker found that Lathrop was in really poor shape.

Dr. Parker told me, "He was begun on chelation therapy in late September. After his seventh treatment it became unnecessary for Lathrop to continue on his vast collection of drugs. He was taken off the medications that he had been taking prior to the chelation treatments. In their place, the patient was put on a nutritional program with vitamin and mineral supplements, which is all a part of the chelation program."

After the man had received thirty-four intravenous injections with EDTA, he was feeling tremendously better and had a lot more energy. He found himself walking long distances just for the sake of getting some exercise, which is also a part of the chelation program. Lathrop mowed the grass in his entire Texas-size yard. He dug holes for fence posts, lifted and strained in heavy work around the house, and finally decided that it was time to return to an income-producing occupation. Now Lathrop works a full twelve-hour day, six days a week, and never feels any chest pain. He was retested by Dr. Parker, and the current results showed significant improvement over his baseline test readings. His blood pressure is now normal.

Thanks to chelation therapy, the man is able to live a more active and productive life. Lathrop returns once a month to Dr. Parker for some maintenance chelation therapy and to have his health progress recorded. He is doing fine.

CHAPTER SIX
The Safety and Possible Side Effects of Chelation Therapy

Adrian Milford LaDeau of Canon City, Colorado, is the patient of chelating physician, James R. Fish, M.D., who is medical director of the Springs Medical Preventics Clinic in Colorado Springs, Colorado. Mr. LaDeau has written a letter for publication and distributes it to anyone he hears of who suffers with a disease connected in some way to hardening of the arteries. He is exceedingly enthusiastic about chelation therapy, which he testifies to having surely saved his life.

You see, prior to coming under the care of Dr. Fish, the patient was seen by famous Texas heart surgeon Denton Cooley, M.D., and also by a few protégés of Michael E. DeBakey, M.D., of the Baylor University College of Medicine in Houston. Dr. DeBakey, during 1966, designed an artificial heart device for patients who have to undergo open heart operations for replacement of heart valves although they are poor surgical risks. In Dr. DeBakey's estimation, these patients have such severely diseased cardiac systems that they could not tolerate the operation without some temporary assistance to the functioning of their hearts during the early postoperative period. The DeBakey heart-assist machine can be installed only by means of open heart surgery. It is attached half in and half outside of the chest wall and is designed for no more than temporary use. Dr. Gallagher, one of Dr. Debakey's protégés, told Mr.

LaDeau that he was very close to death and required a heart transplant.

The following is what Adrian LaDeau explains to people in his letter: "'A heart transplant is your only chance to live.' That is what I was told in Houston in March 1982 after [sustaining] a severe heart attack.

"My surgical experience began in 1979 when an angiogram showed two arteries blocked and the third was 15 percent open. I had a triple bypass and in seven months they [the three coronary artery graphs] had all closed off. So many vessels were involved and a portion of the heart missing in the first surgery that they [the surgeons] couldn't go back in. Heart attacks and angina continued and I began to have memory lapses, headaches, speech problems, and weakness. After the severe attack in March 1982, my DeBakey-trained team said no other treatment was available and that 'everything is over unless you opt for a transplant. You otherwise *might* live until August.'

"I went to the library [in the hospital] and checked the literature on transplants. No one who had a heart transplant for arteriosclerosis had ever lived more than two years, so I checked out of the hospital and asked for a second opinion given by Dr. Denton Cooley of the Texas Heart Institute [in Houston]. Dr. Cooley also believed a transplant was my only hope, but I again declined.

"I moved to Colorado and found Dr. Fish at the Springs Medical Preventics Clinic in Colorado Springs who offered chelation therapy. I had previously heard about this therapy but when I asked my Houston doctors about it they advised me not to waste my time and money.

"I have noticed feeling better in every way since about the second session of chelation therapy. I have no more problem with chest pains and have not taken nitroglycerine for quite a while. My exercise tolerance has improved from zero to walking three miles a day. I have no more headaches and only occasionally do I have the flashing lights in my vision. I am more alert and active and have even started back working in my woodworking shop."

Besides pointing out to the patient that he would be wasting money and time undergoing chelation treatments, one of LaDeau's Texas-based heart surgeons also condemned the therapy as toxic, unsafe, replete with undesirable side effects, and tantamount to committing suicide if he allowed the IV chelating needle to enter his vein. Such statements frequently expounded by members of establishment medicine are blatant falsehoods that come from being misinformed or non-informed or from ignoring the true facts as they have been established by the physicians who use chelation therapy to overcome occlusive vascular disease.

Please be aware that cardiovascular surgeons, chest surgeons, peripheral vascular surgeons, and other members of the health profession who treat heart and blood vessel diseases with establishment medical methods are in direct competition for patients with those maverick physicians who utilize chelation therapy as the preferred procedural technique. As you will learn in Chapter Seven, financial considerations of some physicians' own vested interests are among the factors keeping chelation therapy away from common usage for the American medical consumer.

SOURCES OF DOUBT ABOUT THE SAFETY OF CHELATION THERAPY

Chelation therapy is among the safest of medical treatments. Over 500,000 American patients and about 8 million people in Canada and overseas have received the treatment. Not counting the multimillions of chelation treatments provided to young patients for lead poisoning, approximately 6 million infusions have been administered in the United States just for the reversal of degenerative diseases associated with hardening of the arteries. In the past twelve years of record keeping, not one death has occurred due specifically to chelation therapy when administered by physicians who follow the standard protocol of the American College of Advancement in Medicine.

The record of no chelation therapy mortalities probably goes back to 1954 when, because of experimentation with excessive IV dosages of EDTA, there had been two deaths relating in some way to the treatment. Norman E. Clarke, Sr., M.D., then the director of medical research at the Providence Hospital in Detroit, who did the early work on IV chelation therapy, reported those two cases from among his first EDTA patients. They had been administered up to 10 grams (gm) of EDTA daily, five days a week, within an exceedingly short period of IV administration, which the ACAM protocol now considers a severe overdose. The recommended maximum dosage is currently just 3 grams, given by IV injection only one to three times weekly as a three- to four-hour drip. This is quite a safe program of EDTA administration, according to the meticulous records kept over at least the past decade. I have pointed out earlier in this book that, unfortunately, the opponents of chelation therapy, grasping at any evidence available, and possessing nothing much to condemn about the treatment, still focus on those old 1954 deaths as proof that EDTA administered intravenously can cause harm to the patient.

The scientific truth prevails however: chelation therapy with ethylene diamine tetraacetic acid administered IV is three and a half times safer than taking an aspirin tablet for a headache. The proof comes from EDTA's LD-50 of 2,000 milligrams (mg) per kilogram (kg), in humans. LD-50 stands for the pharmaceutical term "lethal dose 50," the dose of a substance that is fatal to 50 percent of the test animals to which it is administered. The higher the number of milligrams of the substance per kilogram of animal weight able to be administered, the safer the substance. Aspirin, which is acetylsalicylic acid, has an LD-50 of only 558 mg per kg, in humans. It is less than a third as safe as IV EDTA or more oral chelating agents.

Having lived to be 94 years old by keeping himself robust and fit with chelation therapy, the senior Dr. Clarke (who had a chelating physician son, Norman E. Clarke, Jr., M.D.) is credited with originally researching the potential benefits of EDTA and its use in the treatment of occlusive vascular disease. In an article that he wrote for publication in the August 1960 issue of *The American Journal of Cardiology*, Volume II, Number 2, Dr. Clarke said: "For several years we have been administering intravenously to patients with advanced occlusive vascular disease 3 to 5 gm of EDTA."

Please note that in this old paper, published six years later than occurrence of the patient deaths from possible overdosage, Dr. Clarke indicated that he had lowered the IV EDTA dosage. Possibly he did it after experiencing the two sets of complications in medical practice. At first the dose was halved to 5 gm, then it went to 3 gm in 1960 as the optimal dose for a maximum effect. As the officially ACAM recognized safe and efficacious EDTA dose, it has remained 3 gm for more than these past twenty-nine years. And no deaths have been recorded with the reduced IV dosage.

Dr. Clarke continued in his article, "An accumulated experience with several hundred patients has demonstrated that the overall relief from the manifestations of occlusive vascular disease has been superior to that obtained with other methods. In occlusive vascular disease of the brain there has been uniform relief of vertigo, and the signs of senility, even when advanced, have been significantly relieved . . . In summary, the treatment of atherosclerotic vascular complications with the chelating agent EDTA is supported by a large volume of information."

This senior cardiologist and internist reported that he had been able to shrink kidney stones and make them disappear with administering chelation therapy so that the patient could avoid an operation. He said that he took patients having kidneys that were calcified and practically non-functioning and restored them to normal functioning. He had treated a large number of people who were going to accept heart surgery and then changed their minds, choosing chelation therapy as a viable alternative.   Then they never needed heart surgery. Dr. Clarke remarked on his marvelous results using chelation therapy for senility. As it related to safety of administration, the pioneering chelator was convinced that there was no risk. He took chelation therapy himself, twice a month as a life extension tool. After undergoing an initial series of IV injections with EDTA, he continued using chelation therapy for the next thirty-two years.

ANSWERING CONCERNS ABOUT SAFETY

Alfred Soffer, M.D., doesn't agree that chelation therapy with EDTA is safe. In the September 1975 issue of the *Journal of the American Medical Association* (JAMA), Dr. Soffer wrote: "It is mandatory that the physician be familiar with the potential dangers of these powerful agents. The role of chelating agents in the treatment of heavy metal poisoning appears to be secure. Yet to be determined is the ultimate status of chelation in a number of diseases, listed in this volume." Dr. Soffer's quote, inserted in the article in JAMA, was taken from his 1964 book, written for physicians, called *Chelation Therapy*.

As far as this quote is concerned, even today, Soffer says it is still valid. He believes chelating agents are potent medications having long-standing effects that are little understood, inasmuch as they have not been followed for an extended period.

Yet, Garry F. Gordon, M.D., former medical director of Minera-Lab Inc., former president and chairman of the board of directors of ACAM, and the medical consultant for my book, *The Chelation Answer* (M. Evans & Co., 1982, hardcover), points out that chelation therapy has been safe enough to give to toddlers when they have come in contact with lead-based paint. For over twenty years, it has been standard treatment for lead poisoning throughout the United States. The Department of Environmental Medicine of the Mount Sinai School of Medicine of the City University of New York urges the use of IV EDTA in even minimal cases of lead poisoning, because the authorities believe that the danger of any exposure to lead is so great and the safety of the EDTA is so high.

The National Institute for Occupational Safety and Health (NIOSH) has published a pamphlet written by Kenneth Bridbord, M.D., on the dangers of administering chelation therapy for lead toxicity. The pamphlet *Prophylactic Chelation Therapy in Occupational Lead Poisoning: A Review* states: "The potential for chronic administration of chelating agents to cause kidney damage is a special concern. Adverse effects from chelating agents have been observed following both oral and intravenous administration. Both EDTA and penicillamine [another oral chelating agent] have the potential to cause harm. The prevailing medical opinion is strongly opposed to the use of chelating agents on a prophylactic basis [for lead poisoning]. Wherever chelating agents are used, there is a need for close medical supervision, including careful evaluation of renal function. Death and severe injury during and following use of chelating agents have been reported in the medical literature."

Physicians providing their occlusive vascular disease patients with chelation therapy are not the likely objects of this NIOSH warning. There are several differences between antidoting lead poisoning and removing atherosclerotic plaque from clogged arteries.

First, lead is the most toxic of metals and is most likely to cause kidney damage unless there is close monitoring of its removal through the kidney passageways. The lead must go out of the body very slowly so that it won't poison the kidney. There was a time when EDTA had been given by mouth to workers in occupations dealing with lead for overcoming lead poisoning. Combining with lead dust ingested from the work place, orally administered ethylene diamine tetraacetic acid would react in the patient's stomach and be more easily absorbed. Instead of eliminating the lead, therefore, the oral EDTA actually increased the amount of toxicity. Although the members of ACAM had not recommended that physicians prescribe taking EDTA orally, their position has since changed. Garry Gordon claims that when EDTA is taken orally, it acts as a chelating agent and has beneficial effects.

Second, poison control centers giving children chelation therapy for ingestion of lead administer the treatment a minimum of three times a week, while it is standard ACAM protocol procedure to treat vascular patients on the average only about twice a week.

Third, orally administered penicillamine is a much more toxic agent than infused EDTA. While penicillamine is frequently employed to overcome the symptoms of rheumatoid arthritis, it is definitely more toxic than ethylene diamine tetraacetic acid.

The California Medical Association (CMA) still worries about possible dangers to a chelated patient's kidneys. This worry exists, despite the published works of Drs. McDonagh, Rudolph, and Cheraskin, which statistically show IV EDTA improving their patient's impaired kidney function. Apparently, the CMA is unaware of these documented studies. So, failing to catch up with the newest chelation therapy research, the CMA continues to hark back to another old case of a chelated patient with kidney problems.

The case involved a former Anaheim, California, physician named Rudolf Alsleben, M.D., a brilliant maverick who had been bringing patients some remarkable controls for their various health problems. A young woman who Dr. Alsleben had been treating claimed that her kidney failure was a direct cause of chelation therapy. The personal injury suit she brought against the doctor following her eventual recovery found the jury ruling in the patient's favor. Then the CMA revoked Dr. Alsleben's medical license, not for utilizing chelation therapy for an unapproved application but for using poor medical judgment and negligent practice procedures.

Biotoxicologist Bruce W. Halstead, M.D., who had testified in that medical malpractice case on behalf of chelation therapy rather than in defense of the physician, explained how the defendant failed to test the patient for kidney functioning. Dr. Halstead said,

"Dr. Alsleben didn't do his job; he didn't do his homework, and there was no way you could defend the guy."

The woman had taken over 200 intravenous injections with EDTA and half the time never even saw the doctor. She would visit the office, plop herself into an easy chair, roll up her sleeve, and the nurse slipped in the needle. Inasmuch as the patient was the victim of juvenile diabetes with a history of kidney impairment, Dr. Alsleben probably was rendering awfully inappropriate medical care. Her abundant health problems made careful monitoring absolutely imperative. Interesting to note that the young woman had some kind of charitable arrangement by which she never paid Dr. Alsleben a penny for the chelation treatment.

The enemies of chelation therapy point to the Alsleben incident as evidence of therapeutic hazard with injecting EDTA. It's not a hazard, of course, but rather indicates that any chelating physician needs to be ACAM-trained and certified. He or she must be conversant with the latest advances around the country being discovered almost daily by the treatment's dispensers. The chelator must be a user of non-invasive testing procedures and tailor each chelating agent administration to fit the individual's requirements. The rules of administration have been laid down in the chelation therapy certification regulations proposed and administered by the American Board of Chelation Therapy.

THE AMERICAN BOARD OF CHELATION THERAPY (ABCT)

In the early part of 1977, physician members of the American College of Advancement in Medicine (ACAM) realized that chelation therapy was rapidly becoming a well-defined subspecialty of medicine. It became imperative for those physicians who had expertise and knowledge in the treatment to participate in teaching and instructing their colleagues in this new form of therapy, including its benefits, proper use, applications, administration, contraindications, and precautions. Teaching programs in chelation therapy were established in which more experienced doctors in this field could relate their findings and knowledge.

It soon became apparent that some distinction was needed to recognize those physicians possessing, either through practice, experience, and/or study, more extensive knowledge about the chelation process and its chemistry. Initial attempts were made by ACAM to establish a certifying program for recognizing the learned doctor in this new area of specialty medicine. During the following years a program of education and certification functioned, but without good definition or organization.

In 1981, a separate certifying organization comprised of physicians recognized by their peers as being chelation therapy experts was appointed by ACAM. The original founding board members spent a year holding discussions and finally adopted a constitution and bylaws for an autonomous non-profit, educational organization known as the American Board of Chelation Therapy (ABCT) with offices located at 70 West Huron Street, Chicago, Illinois 60610; telephone (312) 787-ABCT. William Mauer, D.O., is the ABCT board chairman and Jack Henck is executive director.

ABCT is recognized by the American Board of Medical Specialties as the certifying board in the subspecialty of chelation therapy. The requirements for physician certification as a chelation therapy specialist necessitate the candidate holding either a doctor of osteopathy (D.O.) or doctor of medicine (M.D.) degree and that he or she currently be licensed to practice medicine in the state in which the candidate practices. Two letters recommending the candidate to ABCT are required from any two physicians who have attained diplomate status in chelation therapy. He or she files an application with ABCT to take the written examination composed of 100 true and false and multiple-choice questions on the computer-generated test. Prior to being tested, the candidate should study the ABCT teaching materials and must attend an ABCT-sponsored series of workshops.

Upon successfully completing the written test, a candidate becomes eligible to take the oral examination before his peers. The actual oral examination however must be preceded by submitting a certified affidavit stating that he or she has been responsible for administering not less than 1,000 chelation treatments to patients under his or her direct responsibility and control. Also necessary to be submitted to ABCT preceding the oral examination are copies of six complete chelated patient records having at least six months of follow-up examinations and appraisal of therapy under the candidate's direct responsibility and control. These six patient records must be presented in the documented, organized format suggested by ABCT.

With his or her application to take the oral examination, the candidate must also submit a minimum of ten referenced questions with their answers acceptable to the examination committee of the board for use in its data bank for future written examinations. These ten questions must adhere to the format of prior examinations. The candidate must also submit evidence of his or her having completed the preceptorship training requirements for chelation therapy as outlined in the current protocol for preceptorship.

After the candidate has completed the various pretest requirements, he or she will then be allowed to take the oral examination before his or her professional peers. Upon successful completion of the exam, the candidate will be proposed for ABCT certification as diplomate.

Objectives and goals of ABCT include defining the specific area of medicine within its jurisdiction. Strictly for the candidate physicians, it establishes teaching workshops; provides reading and study material in the forms of books, articles, and pamphlets; and produces educational materials such as audio and video learning tools. The board administers a series of testing procedures as comprehensive and unbiased as possible. Its testing procedures have been created through the use of a computer data system allowing computer generation of test questions and grading of these questions. Finally, after the candidate has satisfactorily completed all of the ABCT requirements, it bestows the status of diplomate, recognizing the doctor as a trained expert in the field of chelation therapy. Continued recognition of this status is maintained through a process of recertification and reexamination every five years.

IS CHELATION THERAPY REALLY SAFE?

In answering the question, "Is chelation therapy really safe?" it is necessary for you to realize that all chemical agents can be toxic if used in large enough quantities or high enough dosages. Plain drinking water is unsafe if you take in more than you can assimilate. Thus, EDTA chelation therapy could be made unsafe by giving it incorrectly. Incorrect administration means not following the protocol set forth by the ACAM and its teaching arm, the ABCT.

Dr. Bruce Halstead explains in *The Scientific Basis of EDTA Chelation Therapy* that "when EDTA chelation therapy is properly administered by a well-trained physician and nursing staff, it is one of the safest major therapeutic modalities available in the chronic degenerative disease armamentarium. It is also one of the most rewarding therapies for both the patient and the medical staff because of the beneficial results produced."

Oral chelating agents, which will be described in Part Two, starting with Chapter Nine, may be considered safe when the dosages and periodical intake recommended by the manufacturer are closely followed. I make this statement predicated on the product safety examination each manufacturer had to go through when submitting his nutritional ingredients for inspection by the appropriate U.S. or foreign governmental agencies. If such inspections have not been carried out, the oral chelating agent should not be considered safe for human consumption. How do you know if the product has been checked by the United States, Canadian, Japanese, West German, British, or other country-of-origin's Food and Drug Administration (FDA)? Request that information from the product maker. Get the statement in writing, if you are doubtful. Severe penalties are the consequences for a pharmaceutical or nutrient manufacturer if lies on this important matter are disseminated.

As safety for human use is related to ethylene diamine tetraacetic acid (EDTA), it had better be safe inasmuch as the substance has totally permeated Western industrialized society and has gone well into the Third World countries. There is likely never a day that you or I don't have direct contact with EDTA, taking it into our bodies in some form. The FDA allows its inclusion in photographic agents, organic systems, rubber fabrics, textiles, water softeners, emulsifiers, germicides, leather goods, decontaminants, cloth fabrics, hair dyes, cosmetics, fungicides, flavorings, soft drinks, salad dressings, herbicides, plant foods, frozen vegetables, paper, metal cleaners, soaps, detergents, bath oils, hair waving lotions, canned goods, stabilizers, beer, pharmaceuticals, common foods, facial creams, suntan oils, and much more. You probably ingest EDTA at every meal. You are likely to bathe in it, put it on your lips, rub it in your hair, sip it in your cocktail, work with it, color with it, kill bugs with it, sterilize your skin with it, clean with it, make yourself beautiful with it, and do a great deal more with it. The average person probably takes into his body more than the equivalent of one milligram of EDTA per kilogram of body weight per day and suffers no ill effects from it. (A 150-pound person weighs approximately 70 kilograms.) EDTA is a remarkably safe substance for human beings, and we have put it to work in society for our personal convenience and welfare.

EDTA not only evades toxicity to human beings, it actually detoxifies calcium, lead, copper, and other heavy metals from your body. A fine example of how this substance works to detoxify the body was presented to the ACAM by Durk Pearson, co-author of *Life Extension* (Warner Books, 1982, hardcover). Mr. Pearson said: "Did you ever take a good look at a package of frozen brussels sprouts? They are so intensely bright green you would think they had been dyed with some sort of green dye. They seem unnaturally green. In fact, the brussels sprouts are not dyed. That green is just good old ordinary chlorophyll. You are seeing chlorophyll that has not been auto-oxidized. When chlorophyll gets auto-oxidized it turns brown like brown leaves in the fall. Heme [as the hemoglobin in the blood] turns brown too. Heme and chlorophyll are similar substances. Heme has iron and chlorophyll has magnesium, but both are comprised of heme groups. They turn brown upon oxidizing.

"The reason that the brussels sprouts look so green," Durk Pearson continued, "is that they are washed with a solution of EDTA and citric acid [both chelating agents] to remove the iron and copper that would otherwise be contaminants on the leaves from the soil and the fertilizer. With the iron and copper being removed there is so much less free radical damage to the brussels sprouts' leaves that they stay crisp, hard, fresh, and bright green. If the brussels sprouts had not been washed with the chelating agents, you would find yourself with brown, limp brussels sprouts even though you had just taken them from the deep freeze. The reason that most frozen vegetables [broccoli, green beans, string beans, etc.] have this incredible bright green color is that they have been given chelation therapy. Give the brussels sprouts chelation therapy and they will have a very much extended life span."

People react in the same way to chelation therapy as do Brussels sprouts. With chelation therapy as part of their lifestyle, people don't form brown liver spots on the skin as they grow older; they grow older more slowly and have their life expectancies extended.

Like any other food or drug, each of the oral or intravenous chelating agents are capable of producing some sort of a biological effect, depending on the dosage ingested. The chelating foods will tend to have a relatively mild effect and thus work more slowly for an individual. The injectable chelator will produce a generally more pronounced and predictable effect. The injectables have a toxic range largely more controlled by established dosage levels. Injectable chelating agents are known to produce a much faster effect, usually for the better in a sick person, than oral chelating agents. In Chapter Nine, I shall be more specific about the speed with which oral chelating agents work.

The National Institute for Occupational Safety and Health in another of the agency's 1976 publications, "Registry of Toxic Effects of Chemical Substances," has defined a toxic substance as "one that demonstrates the potential to induce cancer, tumors, or neoplastic effects in human or experimental animals; to induce a permanent transmissible change in the characteristics of an offspring from those of its human or experimental animal parents; to cause the production of physical defects in the developing human or experimental animal embryo; to produce death in experimental or domestic animals exposed via the respiratory tract, skin, eyes, mouth, or other routes; to produce irritation or sensitization of the skin, eyes, or respiratory passages; to diminish mental alertness, reduce motivation, or alter behavior of humans; to adversely affect the health of a normal or disabled person of any age or of either sex by producing reversible or irreversible bodily injury or by endangering life or causing death from exposure via the respiratory tract, skin, eye, mouth, or any other route in any quantity, concentration, or dose reported for any length of time."

EDTA and most other oral and injectable chelating agents are similar to various other chemical substances in that their toxic effects are governed by fundamental toxicological principles. They are not more toxic than other common chelating ingredients present in nature. In therapeutics, the recommended chelating agents are mostly of a mild and innocuous nature and do not bring on toxic responses under usual conditions of use.

The safety of EDTA intravenous administration for the removal of serum ionic calcium is assured, for the actual toxicity of EDTA varies with the metal chelate that is formed. Calcium EDTA is safe when formed in human blood vessels inasmuch as 95 percent of it gets excreted through the kidney tubules and the other 5 percent goes through the liver and out the intestinal tract exceedingly fast. EDTA is not metabolized in the body. Its biological half-life is about one hour. Within a twenty-four-hour period, an infusion of this amino acid sees 99 percent of it gone from the body with just half of 1 percent remaining after forty-eight hours. Because of possible precipitation by the gastric juice, EDTA is destroyed in the stomach.

THE AMERICAN COLLEGE OF ADVANCEMENT IN MEDICINE (ACAM)

Chelating agents that have already been or will come to be described here are not known as producing toxic responses in human beings when the agents, oral or injectables, are ingested at ACAM recommended dosage levels, accepted intervals of administration, and usual speeds of absorption. If you have technical questions relating to chelation therapy's safety, side effects, administration, physiology, benefits, patient candidates, chelating physician locations, or anything else concerning degenerative disease or cardiovascular disease treatment, my suggestion is that you should contact the American College of Advancement in Medicine Inc., Edward A. Shaw, Ph.D., Executive Director. The ACAM is located at 23121 Verdugo Drive, #204, Laguna Hills, California 92653; telephone in California (714) 583-7666, outside California (800) 532-3688.

The ACAM is a nationwide, traditionally trained group of physicians who have formally adopted EDTA chelation therapy as their standard method of medical treatment for patients they find are suffering from occlusive vascular disease involving the cerebral, coronary, or peripheral circulation. Occlusive vascular disease is for all practical purposes generally synonymous with the terms "hardening of the arteries" and "arteriosclerosis," but may include other causes of blocked blood flow, including spasm and loss of compliance and elasticity of blood vessels due to the accumulation of calcium as seen in the aging process.

ACAM physicians spend their resources to investigate the scientific evidence regarding chelation therapy and any other major substitute, newly evolving treatments. The organization has developed a written protocol with complete guidelines for the appropriate, careful, effective, and safe application of EDTA chelation therapy. Its members are required to adhere to this protocol and all of its reporting requirements. ACAM members are offered the opportunity to become recognized as specialists in chelation therapy by obtaining the diplomate status as bestowed on them by the American Board of Chelation Therapy. As I described earlier, attaining diplomate status comes only from extensive study, with appropriate written and oral examinations and clinical experience requirements (see also appendix).

The college now has over 400 members in the United States, comprising M.D.'s and D.O.'s. Many of the major subspecialties in medicine are represented among the membership including internal medicine, cardiology, vascular surgery, pharmacology, physical chemistry, ophthalmology, orthopedic surgery, biotoxicology, and others. The members bring a broad vista of expertise to ACAM study groups, forums, conferences, and seminars.

The American College of Advancement in Medicine does not represent all of the chelating physicians in the United States. There are probably well over 1,000 American doctors who utilize chelation therapy to a greater or lesser degree in the treatment of arteriosclerosis. ACAM records indicate that about 500,000 Americans have taken chelation treatment, but it's likely that more than one million patients is a more realistic figure. Non-members do not have to report their treatment schedules into the ACAM statistical bank. Members usually do. This vast clinical experience has provided the College with an unparalleled opportunity to observe the short- and long-term effects of chelation therapy in all forms of occlusive vascular disease. The records show that about 82 percent of chelated patients show distinct improvement, both subjectively and objectively, as a result of their treatment program.

With all of this treatment history, chelation therapy has shown itself to be absolutely safe. When the ACAM protocol for proper application has been adhered to, not a single documented instance of a patient's death as a direct response of the application of EDTA chelation therapy has occurred since 1954. Still, since the organization is in existence just slightly more than twelve years but was in its formative stages two years before that, ACAM points to merely fourteen years of safety for chelation therapy.

Member physicians of the ACAM believe it is unfair to patients who are attempting to get true information regarding all possible cardiovascular disease treatment alternatives not to receive chelation therapy information. They are sick people, in many cases attempting to avoid proposed peripheral vascular surgery (including amputation) and chest surgery (including coronary artery bypass). In other circumstances the inquiring persons may be sons and daughters or spouses looking for a way other than commitment of their elderly senile family members to rest homes, drugs, and other forms of treatment. All too often medical consumers are not told about chelation therapy by their family physicians who are practicing in the medical mainstream. Lack of information, in most instances, comes from the family doctors themselves knowing little or nothing about chelation treatment. Patients seeking help for their occlusive vascular disease must be given at least the choice of contacting the ACAM to receive the information required. They cannot and are not given chelation therapy information from the American Medical Association, the American College of Chest Physicians, or any other professional association representing the vested interests of individual organized medical groups. These groups jealously guard their own profit and are not interested in promoting the widespread utilization and development of this important new treatment. In fact, they are competing with chelation therapists for patient dollars. Vascular surgeons, for instance, become highly concerned for their income when they discover that 82 percent of patients ordinarily coming under the knife no longer need operations. The patients receive instead significant benefits from an alternative therapy that is markedly decreasing the number of surgical procedures for vascular disease in this country.

POSSIBLE SIDE EFFECTS OF CHELATION THERAPY

Even with all the physiological benefits offered the individual from taking chelation therapy in oral or intravenous form, however, the treatment is not devoid of possible side effects. There are certain precautions to follow with receiving EDTA infusions or going on your own into oral chelating mechanisms. If you know the possible side effects of treatment, you will exercise the common sense precautions that come naturally to any thinking individual.

First, you must recognize that serum-ionizable calcium levels are immediately reduced with intravenous EDTA and only over the long term eventually reduce with slower acting oral chelating agents.

Second, the medical literature warns doctors that it is possible for improper administration of IV EDTA through excessive dosage or too rapid a rate of injection to induce certain serious symptoms such as spasm and twitching of muscles (tetany), particularly those of the face, hands, and feet. Such tetany is caused by a reduction in the blood calcium level. Other serious symptoms that chelating physicians are cautioned about are convulsions, severe cardiac arrhythmias (irregular heartbeats), and even respiratory arrest in which case the patients' lack of breathing could bring on death. These are the worst possible risks of EDTA infusion, particularly when the solution is dripped too quickly or the dosage is well over three grams.

The very serious symptoms that I have just described are extremely rare or just don't happen. They are mentioned here because they could happen. Instead, when appropriate precautions are taken by the supervising doctor during IV administration, adequate mobilization of calcium from the body's calcium stores does occur, which then corrects the condition of induced hypocalcemia (lack of serum calcium). This mobilization of extracirculatory calcium is mediated, as I have described earlier, through the parathyroid gland, which responds to the EDTA blood stream action, by markedly increased parathormone release. Parathormone is the hormone that goes to the metastatic calcium deposited in the hardened arteries, the kidney stones, the bursae, the arthritic joints, or in other places and pulls it out of those deposits to replace the missing serum ionic calcium.

Note: If your parathyroid gland is going to respond correctly to chelation therapy, you must have an adequate intake of dietary magnesium plus the absence in your body of parathyroid beta blockers such as Inderal and parathyroids that are healthy.

Of the various adverse reactions possibly seen by the doctor with occasional administrations of EDTA chelation therapy, the most serious that could appear are hypotension, hypoglycemia, and hypocalcemia. Hypotension is a drop in blood pressure. Hypoglycemia is a reduction in blood sugar levels. Hypocalcemia is an acute lowering of the amount of ionic calcium in the blood.

For people who have high blood pressure as a disease symptom, temporary hypotension may be advantageous. One of the first disease conditions to be normalized by chelation therapy is hypertension. For those patients who experience a lowering of blood sugar when taking IV EDTA, some nutritional intake during the four-hour infusions, such as a banana, a sandwich, or other food, tends to lessen the hypoglycemic reaction. You should have eaten immediately before the infusion, but avoid consuming foods that are high in calcium such as dairy products. For someone showing signs of hypocalcemia, the doctor keeps ready in the chelation administration area a syringe filled with calcium solution for fast intravenous injection.

Other possible adverse reactions that have been reported to the ACAM as part of its monitoring and record-keeping procedures are: pain or burning at the site of infusion that is overcome by adding magnesium or procaine to the infusion solution, transient numbness around the mouth and lips, mild fever, chills, slight anemia, elevated amounts of sugar in the urine (glycosuria), an abnormally high concentration of uric acid in the blood (hyperuricemia), red skin patches, a flaking skin eruption, and other types of dermatological lesions. These various signs and symptoms are uncommon and are easily reversed as a result of the chelating physician's ACAM training.

In its protocol, the College also reports on other rare side effects of intravenous EDTA injections including headache, thirst, fatigue, muscle cramps, muscle weakness, back pain, numbness, malaise (a general unwell feeling), lassitude (a feeling of weariness), and thrombophlebitis, which may occur with any intravenous fluid infusion. Some gastrointestinal symptoms that you could feel are nausea, vomiting, diarrhea, abdominal cramps, and loss of appetite. Also slipped into the protocol to cover all possible eventualities are cautions about insulin shock, possible calcium embolization, digitalis antagonism effect on the heart, and damage to the reticuloendothelial system with hemorrhagic manifestations following really high doses of EDTA.

Other than severe hypocalcemia, the most serious potential hazard of EDTA infusion that the chelating doctor gets cautioned against is nephrotoxicity, which has been associated with excessive doses of the drug that I reported on earlier as Dr. Clarke's cases. A nephrotoxic substance is something that is poisonous to the kidney. Drs. McDonagh, Rudolph, and Cheraskin have shown that EDTA is not nephrotoxic. (See Chapters Four and Five.) There might be the coexistence of heavy metal toxicity so that lead nephrosis (kidney malfunction) could mistakenly be attributed to the EDTA infusion.

POSSIBLE NEPHROTOXICITY IN CHELATION THERAPY

Heavy metals themselves are a source of kidney poisoning (nephrotoxicity), particularly when the heavy metal is being eliminated through the kidney. This happens even while the lead, mercury, cadmium, nickel, copper, arsenic, antimony, or other heavy metal is bound to EDTA. Therefore, lead EDTA is much more toxic than calcium EDTA. Too rapid an infusion with EDTA could produce an apparent independent nephrotoxicity, which is something the medical establishment is quite fearful of. Orthodox medicine has reason to fear nephrotoxicity, because the majority of traditionally trained physicians have taken no training from the ACAM for EDTA administration. Without such skills, establishment doctors should be worried about causing their chelation patients' nephrotoxicity. Such untrained physicians don't have the rudiments of safety as part of their guidelines.

Besides nephrotoxicity, other urinary symptoms such as the urgency to urinate, nocturia (the passage of urine at night), polyuria (the production of excess quantities of urine), dysuria (difficult or painful urination), oliguria (the production of an abnormally small amount of urine), proteinuria (the presence of protein in the urine), as well as the presence of microscopic casts and cells in the urine have been reported following IV EDTA. There have been sparse reports also of kidney insufficiency, kidney failure, and one report of acute tubular necrosis. Blood has been seen in the urine immediately after chelation therapy, where unsuspected bladder disease such as early cancer was later revealed at examination with a cystoscope.

With all the possibilities of kidney damage or nephrotoxicity from administering EDTA injections, symptoms or signs suggesting nephrotoxicity are usually readily reversed and clear from the patient within a few days after the medication is discontinued. Nevertheless, the chelating physician is trained to assess the patient's kidney function before he or she infuses with EDTA. Periodic blood-urea-nitrogen testing and/creatinine clearance determinations, along with regular urinalyses, are performed during chelation therapy.

The ACAM recommends that chelating physicians begin with diminished doses of EDTA, as little as a half to one gram for the first treatment and gradually work up to the full dose, as calculated by body weight, depending on the patient's tolerance. In addition, prescreening of patients for possible increased body burden of heavy metals through the use of hair and blood analyses helps the doctor identify those having an increased potential for developing nephrosis. Sometimes the chelator carries out provocative twenty-four-hour urine tests for heavy metal intoxication, particularly when such testing is needed to establish a conclusive diagnosis of lead or other metal poisoning.

Patients who have a marginally functioning pair of kidneys are treated with extreme caution by the chelating physician. Regular and frequent evaluations of kidney status are carried out. It is important to recognize that in the past, the potential for nephrotoxicity from chelation therapy was exaggerated by the uninformed majority of the medical profession. Previously pathologists made this mistake because the vacuoles present in the kidney immediately following IV EDTA are a physiological process of pinocytosis. Pinocytosis is the phenomenon sometimes seen in the kidney tubules of folds or invaginations in the surface of the cell membranes to form fluid-filled vesicles. The pathologists thought that the pinocytosis was a sign of toxicity, but it is not. The pinocytosis reverses upon allowing the kidney tissues adequate time between infusions. That is why EDTA is not infused every day.

The experience of the College members to date has been that many patients with even significantly impaired kidney function have been safely treated with intravenous EDTA for their occlusive vascular diseases. Most patients will show subsequent improvement in their initially impaired kidneys. Their renal function tests become normal, since vascular disease of the kidney frequently may be the cause of the impairment. Clear away the arteriosclerosis in the kidney and the organ will function better. A thousand cases of kidney impairment are now documented in files held by the American College of Advancement in Medicine showing that cautious, low-dose, infrequent EDTA infusions, given over a prolonged interval of six to eight hours while adequate high fluid intake is maintained, have produced satisfactory resolution of the patient's vascular disease process with the simultaneous secondary benefit of improving kidney function. Under kidney function testing, the patient will show lower serum creatinine and blood urea nitrogen test readings with increased creatinine clearance.

CHELATION THERAPY ELIMINATES HEART PACEMAKERS

Not only does chelation therapy restore malfunctional kidneys to near normal, the treatment also allows patients with weakened heart muscles to rid themselves of heart pacemaker machines. A pacemaker is a scientific electrical instrument that controls the normal rhythm of the heartbeat when the physiological mechanism fails. It is implanted in the chest and attached to the ventricle by a wire passed through the connecting veins. With the pacemaker installed, the heart rate can be maintained at a steady number of beats per minute, in accordance with what is normal for the individual who is the victim of a damaged heart muscle.

At age 66, Damon Matlock of Clovis, New Mexico, suffered with a damaged heart muscle. Because his heart rate was so irregular, he had a heart pacemaker installed into his chest wall in February 1981.

Now, Mr. Matlock had a long history of circulation problems throughout his body. Surgeons had wanted to do surgery on his carotid arteries, for instance, but could not perform the operation because these arteries in his neck were too occluded. An angiogram had shown less than 5 percent blood flow through the carotids. As a result of such occlusive vascular disease, the man suffered a stroke in September 1981. It left him partially paralyzed. Slurred speech and paralysis on the right side of his body prevented him from getting around or talking well.

In November 1981 Matlock visited John T. Taylor, D.O., and Gerald M. Parker, D.O., at the Doctors Clinic in Amarillo, Texas, to begin chelation therapy as a rehabilitative method for his stroke symptoms. At that time the patient was wearing his pacemaker as usual. Drs. Parker and Taylor performed an extensive blood work-up series of tests along with two circulatory evaluations, a plethys-mography examination, and a Doppler ultrasound differential. The plethysmograph showed left and right carotid arteries to be harden-ing with little elasticity and no pulse regularity.

Matlock was advised by the chelating physicians to take from thirty to sixty intravenous injections with EDTA and to go on the oral chelation agent program. While the patient was taking the treatments, his wife noticed that he was speaking more coher-ently—his words came out plainer. Then he started to use his right arm, which had been affected by the stroke. By the time Matlock had received fifty chelation treatments, his recovery had advanced so much that his physicians felt he could stop the twice weekly infusions and go onto a maintenance program. Drs. Taylor and Parker put him on a schedule of injection boosters every two months. They repeated the plethysmography examination and found that his carotid arteries showed much more uniformity to their beat and more elasticity. Matlock could now talk in long under-standable sentences and could use his right arm rather well.

The most dramatic changes included his ability to move quickly and effectively while maintaining a uniform heart rate, even with the pacemaker turned off. Matlock therefore decided that he could do without his artificial heart machine lying useless under his skin. The patient had the pacemaker removed from his chest wall and no longer experiences chest pain or irregular heartbeats. Matlock's heart is beating properly by itself. Matlock's chelation therapy was responsible for eliminating his need for any heart pacemaker.

CHAPTER SEVEN
Medical Politics and Media Abuse of Chelation Therapy

A television station located in Salt Lake City, Utah, seeking to build audience appeal during the early part of 1979, decided to produce an exposé-type of documentary on "medical quackery." Predominantly Mormon, Salt Lake City's residents seem uniquely blessed with relatively good health as a result of their excellent nutritional practices and their non-drinking and non-smoking lifestyles. Realizing that finding medical charlatanism would be no easy task among the healthy populace, the TV talent people required some expert advice. They therefore approached the city's supposedly authoritative politicians in organized medicine to select an appropriate target. And the finger of condemnation was pointed at chelation therapy, particularly as it was practiced by a leading Salt Lake City exponent of the treatment.

An osteopathic physician, Robert B. Vance, D.O., a former first vice president of the American College of Advancement in Medicine, runs a thriving chelation therapy practice. Dr. Vance is knowledgeable on the subject since he has been an instructor at the College's teaching seminars, is a diplomate in chelation therapy, and is certified by the ABCT. Also, he is co-author of the most complete medical journal article ever published on the intravenous administration of ethylene diamine tetraacetic acid (written by Garry F. Gordon, M.D., and Robert B. Vance, D.O., "EDTA Chelation Therapy for Arteriosclerosis: History and Mechanisms of

Action." Osteopathic Annals 4:38-62, February 1976). The television producers set up their operation to penetrate Dr. Vance's medical practice and use against him anything they could twist in favor of an exciting program. Their intent was to hook an audience into watching the TV station's broadcasts.

I acquired most of the information you are about to read during an investigative journalism trip to Salt Lake City in the summer of 1982.

The plot was planned; the drama cast. Unknown to Dr. Vance, he was assigned the part of villain; his believing patients, whom the TV commentator designated innocent victims, were shown sacrificing their bodies to a treatment labelled fake and dangerous. The heroine's role was given to a 38-year-old actress employed by the TV station who presented herself to Dr. Vance as a patient in need of chelation therapy, to expose him later as a charlatan because supposedly she had nothing wrong with her body. The TV station, KUTV, Channel 2, had apparently been advised by medical politicians that this physician ran a chelation therapy mill.

The woman, acting as a decoy, visited Dr. Vance complaining of angina-like chest pains. Her symptoms were frequent, she lied, affirming that they came on with stress or exertion. The producers' intention was to get the doctor to give chelation therapy to their decoy when the woman did not need it. Then they would reveal the "shocking truth."

Prior to sending their employee to the chelating physician, Channel 2-TV had her examined by a board-certified internist who specializes in kidney disorders (nephrology). This traditional physician is not a friend of the osteopath. According to the patient, the internist allegedly gave her a clean bill of health, although of course she presented him with no symptoms at all to investigate. Unfortunately, the actress failed to completely comprehend exactly what the examination uncovered, and the producers' interpretation of her health status was incorrect. The subsequent error turned out costly for Dr. Vance.

It appears the internist actually found the patient did exhibit diagnostic signs of valvular heart disease. His records show that he had informed her of a "midsystolic click" heard over her heart and even explained that if she had been feeling any anginal symptoms, he would have tested her much more extensively. This information came to the surface much later, when the three-member Board of Osteopathic Examiners of the State of Utah took testimony in a hearing to remove the osteopathic medical license of Robert B. Vance, D.O., because he eventually did administer chelation therapy to the woman, twelve months after the first consultation.

The internist-nephrologist testified at Dr. Vance's hearing that he had told the woman that this heart sound might well represent a partial prolapse of one of the leafs of her mitral valve. He stated that she was informed by him that she must take antibiotics with every dental extraction or upper respiratory infection to guard against the potential of subacute bacterial endocarditis. The internist even testified that the absence of chest pain and other cardiovascular symptoms caused him not to recommend additional heart studies, such as an echocardiogram for possible heart chamber enlargement. He thought that even blood flow studies, including heart catheterization (an angiogram) for pressure differential, was in order to further identify the potential extent of the patient's possible "heart disease." Thus, the internist accepted the woman's negative history and allowed it to help him decide what course of action to follow in managing her case. Since she did not describe any symptoms of chest pain, the specialist did nothing but provide some advice about antibiotics, and let her go.

After almost a year of seeing Dr. Vance approximately once a month, all the while complaining of chest pain and shortness of breath, but without the physician recommending chelation therapy, the woman and her employers were desperate. Her medical care was getting too costly for the TV station, and they did not yet have an exposé story. Dr. Vance had classified the patient as possibly having symptoms compatible to "cardiac neurosis" and had been merely treating her with good nutrition. He could not do much more. The woman never allowed any non-invasive diagnostic tests because she said she could not afford their extra costs. She also refused to have the standard pelvic examination requested by Dr. Vance.

The patient and her employers were disappointed because they hardly dreamed it would take so long to get her into chelation therapy. They had almost given up the entrapment of Dr. Vance but decided to make a last ditch attempt. She finally brought up the subject of chelation therapy herself and asked him for the treatment. She said that his more conservative nutritional therapies were not doing anything to relieve her chest pain, and she was suffering unnecessarily when Dr. Vance had the means to remove her discomfort.

Inasmuch as he had also discovered the patient's heart valve impairment, Dr. Vance came to the conclusion that chelation therapy might help her indeed. The patient therefore did succeed in getting him to start her on a program of intravenous EDTA injections. It was then that she went on television and told viewers that Dr. Vance had treated her heart without any cause. She said that no heart disease existed and obviously this charlatan had given her chelation therapy just to collect her money.

Channel 2 played their videotaped single interview with Dr. Vance about ten times over the next eighteen months. The commentator declared that this perfectly healthy woman had been chelated strictly for the cash that it brought the doctor.

Not once during the periodic showing of this ongoing exposé TV program did the station employee qualify her statements or explain that she was possibly inaccurate. Never did the woman reveal that she actually suffered from valvular heart disease. Nor did the first nephrologist-internist step forward with true information about the patient, in the event that she didn't know it. The woman gave the impression to Channel 2 that her examining internist had told her she was "perfectly fine," which is apparently what she preferred to believe; otherwise, she could not have gone on television to tell the audience on their evening news program how she had been needlessly treated for a "heart condition" when her heart had been diagnosed as perfect.

Either the patient did not really understand what the internist claims he told her, or he failed to adequately explain it, or perhaps he just forgot to explain it to her. But the internist's records indicate that he did warn the woman. Perhaps she really wanted a chance to play in the great drama of entrapping an incompetent doctor who was treating her for nonexistent heart disease with a "dangerous, unproven remedy called chelation therapy just to make more money for himself." Thus, she simply ignored what the internist told her about her possible mitral leaf prolapse so she could go ahead with the broadcast.

The misled television station put so much pressure on the local governmental agencies to stop "this terrible quack," that finally the licensing board of osteopathic examiners in Utah undertook an expensive, lengthy, "narcotic-agent-type" of investigation into Dr. Vance's practice methods.

Having access to health insurance industry computers, the state's investigators were able to review all the health insurance claim forms filed by most of Dr. Vance's patients, which went back more than twelve years. They contacted these patients to see if anyone could be induced to testify against the "bad" doctor. And the attorney general's detectives were able to turn up some dissatisfied patients, who may be found in every physician's practice, especially those still owing big medical bills to the doctor. Anyone they could locate for whom Dr. Vance had ever filled out a health insurance claim form was interviewed, and that individual was asked to testify against him.

After twenty months of such preparation among 10,000 interviewed patients who had visited Dr. Vance during the prior twelve years, the state of Utah finally gathered thirty-seven prosecution witnesses, some not personally contacted but only listed to pad the complaint. Most of the patient names were obtained from the local health insurance office files. In other cases the patient's previous and/or subsequent doctor was also brought in to testify. The total number of thirty-seven people made an impressive lot, however only eight cases were introduced at the trial and three of those were paid decoys. Utah's attorney general brought charges of medical incompetence and/or negligent practices by Dr. Vance to the osteopathic examining board, and hearings were scheduled. However, other patients appreciative of the doctor's services turned out in impressive numbers to defend him.

Two separate hearings over a six-day period were held to determine the fitness of Dr. Vance to continue in osteopathic medical practice, the final one on February 2, 1981. During the first hearing, the state took four and one-half days to present its case. Dozens of patients wrote letters of support to the local media for him. But almost none of these supportive statements were ever expressed to the public on the electronic media or in the press. Only the more sensational attacks against this chelating physician received extensive coverage. The local orthodox medical professionals were chief among his accusers.

Of the many witnesses appearing at the hearings on behalf of Dr. Vance, 51-year-old Dean Baxter of Houston, Texas, was one of the more persuasive people testifying. He is a prominent public relations counselor for Atlantic Richfield Oil Company. Baxter described how two cardiovascular surgeons had told him in separate consultations three and a half years before that he required a quadruple coronary artery bypass operation or he would soon die. After eschewing surgery and undergoing forty chelation treatments and several booster injections with EDTA since, the man said that he is "now busy and very active in every way." Dr. Vance was the chelating physician who first provided Baxter with his life-saving treatment.

Fifty-year-old Benjamin Christiansen of Salt Lake City, another patient treated by Dr. Vance, had been told by a cardiologist in 1979 that he had less than a year to live. His speedy death from heart attack was assured from the effects of severe hardening of the arteries around the heart. At that time before taking chelation therapy, Christiansen explained to the board of osteopathic examiners, he could not walk two city blocks without experiencing severe angina pain. Upon completing a series of twenty-two intravenous chelation injections, however, Christiansen found that his health and vitality have been restored to the point where he now hikes and rides a snowmobile at every opportunity.

Joyce Walker of the same city, interviewed by the *Salt Lake City Deseret News*, said that she had first sought out Dr. Vance nineteen years before, and later had received nutritional and chelation therapy for several cardiovascular health problems, including hypercalcemia (elevated blood levels of calcium), which other doctors had been unable to adequately diagnose. The treatment completely eliminated her difficulties. Furthermore, Walker told of an added benefit of the chelation therapy. It was responsible for dissolving a kidney stone that had been severely troublesome to her but isn't anymore. The stone is now completely gone.

Some physicians testified on behalf of Dr. Vance, too. A leading chelation therapy specialist and expert on complex gastrointestinal disorders, Michael Gerber, M.D., of Mill Valley, California, described nutritional approaches to degenerative diseases and backed up Dr. Vance on his use of chelation therapy. In an outright display of the abuse of government power, the hearing transcript shows that Utah's prosecuting attorney, Leon Halgren, found Dr. Gerber's testimony so devastating to his case that this prosecutor threatened to turn over a transcript of Dr. Gerber's remarks to the California Medical Association, as if testimony in support of Dr. Vance was itself criminal.

During my visit to the San Francisco metropolitan area on September 26, 1983, I learned that Dr. Gerber's testimony had apparently indeed been transferred to the California medical authorities. He has, since the Vance licensure hearing, been forced to retain San Francisco attorneys to ward off a threat to his own right to continue the practice of medicine in the state of California. The medical bureaucrats are trying to stop him from using alternative health care approaches such as megavitamins, hair analysis, chelation therapy, and other non-standard methods. The California Board of Quality Assurance and the California Board of Medical Examiners are both seemingly using the Vance hearing testimony as evidence against Dr. Gerber. What happens in Utah evidently can affect practice procedures in California.

The Utah State Osteopathic Board of Examiners voted on the spot during that second February 10, 1981 hearing for the removal of Dr. Vance's license. But the next day a compromise was worked out with Utah District Court Judge Dean Conder presiding. Dr. Vance was granted temporary permission to practice until a full hearing could be held to determine if the Utah court system could be used to help in the battle for his medical license. Dr. Vance was told "off the record" by the board that he could probably remain in practice and that they would stop harassing him if he merely refrained from offering chelation therapy, using EDTA. The board members wanted him to employ some other means of chelating his patients, perhaps with intravenous vitamin C.

The examining board also denied him the right to employ certain unorthodox diagnostic techniques, such as applied kinesiology and iridology. Applied kinesiology is therapy localization that identifies faults and dysfunctions in the body that have an effect on the nervous system. It is a diagnostic procedure based on the fact that body language never lies. Iridology, also known as irisdiagnosis, is based on the premise that each organ of the body is represented by an area of the iris in the eye. Charts made to show such areas present the organs with the pupil area corresponding to colors and areas on the iris. Iridological diagnosis can indicate an approaching health crisis in a patient.

Moreover, Dr. Vance was forced to report to the state any patient's name on whom he would make a diagnosis of hypoglycemia. This final ruling appears to be an invasion of the patient's privacy, a break in patient-physician confidentiality, and an infringement on the doctor's medical civil rights.

Because he had just opened a new and expanded health care center, Dr. Vance had unfortunately destroyed a large number of old "inactive" patient records during the move. His rebuttal of the prosecutor's charges was therefore much less effective than it might otherwise have been. For this main reason he did not fully respond to all statements made by the prosecution witnesses. Making such a weak case, Dr. Vance found it necessary to accept the conditions of the compromise. He also had to continue making a living to support his wife and ten children.

Having little choice other than to close down his facility and begin practice elsewhere, Dr. Vance therefore consented to eliminate testing with kinesiology and iridology and to stop administering various alternative forms of chelation therapy such as those oral methods that I describe in Part Two. Yet, his practice is currently very busy because he recently saved the life of a famous Dutch singer by the use of oral and intravenous chelation therapy, using ingredients other than ethylene diamine tetraacetic acid. Now many people from Holland and all around the rest of Europe travel to Salt Lake City for the expert medical assistance offered by Dr. Vance.

The osteopathic examining board wasn't bothering him anymore; no final decision had come down to alter the compromise reached. Dr. Vance was continuing to provide medical care for the patients who seek his services, because of restraining orders granted by the courts while his appeal was pending.

In an interesting legal footnote to this typical oppression of a chelating physician, perhaps all remained quiet for Dr. Vance for another reason. The three-member board of the Utah state osteopathic examiners that had heard the Vance case at the time was possibly illegally constituted. It has been suggested by political opponents of Utah's current governor that one of the three members had not met the residence and professional criteria established by the state to be a member of that board. This important fact was seemingly unnoticed or of no great concern to the lower courts; consequently, Dr. Vance appealed his case to the Utah State Supreme Court. Generally in most states, such an illegally constituted board would entirely invalidate the licensure hearing. This being standard legal procedure, the subsequent Vance osteopathic license revocation decision should have been set aside. Dr. Vance and his patients were anxiously awaiting this ruling.

Then tragedy struck! After a year and a half of coming to a decision, the Utah State Supreme Court upheld the osteopathic board of examiners ruling to revoke the medical license of Robert B. Vance, D.O. The Supreme Court mentioned nothing in the decision about the physician's style of practice and his morality. Rather, it was a strictly technical legal decision. It upheld the revocation order and the illegally constituted board of examiners (according to the Utah statutory code) by stating that the board chairperson, an osteopathic psychiatrist named Katherine Greenwood, D.O., was part of "a de facto committee" already established. And "although not qualified for appointment to the Osteopathic Committee..." read the judges' majority decision, "the revocation had been recommended by the requisite majority of the committee without Dr. Greenwood's vote."

Being rebuffed by the Utah State Supreme Court, Dr. Vance has moved from Utah and relocated his chelation therapy practice in Las Vegas, Nevada. Nevada is a state with more liberal laws for the practice of alternative (complementary) methods of healing, including the use of nutritional therapies. Orthomolecular nutrition and more advanced metabolic techniques are employed by Nevada holistic physicians.

Something other physicians or paraprofessionals who are being harried by similar bureaucratic discipline procedures may learn from Dr. Vance's upsetting experience is that as soon as you begin to be investigated or abused by either a state board of examiners, some professional association peer review committee, any health insurance company, the Food and Drug Administration, or other hostile parties, immediately go to federal court against your oppressors. Once you allow yourself to get locked into the state's administrative procedures, you are forced to exhaust all the existing remedies.

Almost invariably, the hearing committee that acts as prosecutor, judge, jury, and sometimes plaintiff's witness is likely to rule against you.

Distressed health professionals tend to lose sight of an important tool to protect themselves against tyranny from the establishment. The civil rights laws are created to protect minorities from being abused—not only blacks, women, and others that we recognize—but also certain physicians and allied health practitioners. Those in preventive medicine are in such a narrow minority group (especially the chelators who are bucking the medical mainstream). In Dr. Vance's case, being an osteopathic physician, practicing preventive medicine, and using chelation therapy, he is a member of practically the ultimate minority (although he is neither black, Hispanic, nor female).

Dr. Vance has been wronged. The media treated him unfairly in order to build an audience, and the resultant public pressure caused his osteopathic peers to respond. Consequently, this chelating physician is continuing to fight back for restoration of his civil right to practice osteopathic preventive medicine using chelation therapy in the state of Utah.

We can summarize this injustice by quoting from the Utah Supreme Court's minority opinion. Dissenting, Justice Stewart wrote:

> I do not agree that the actions of the representative committee and the district court in this case can be justified on the statutory basis relied upon in the majority opinion, especially when the representative committee was not properly constituted and the appellant did not receive the kind of judicial review in the district court required by statute. Had the representative committee and the Department of Business Regulation promulgated rules governing unprofessional conduct for osteopaths, as contemplated by statute, the case could be remanded for further consideration under those rules. But, because appellant was found guilty of unprofessional conduct on other standards, I submit that the revocation of his license is unconstitutional.

When he walked into his office Monday morning, October 31, 1983, Robert B. Vance, D.O., was forced to remove his framed Utah license to practice osteopathic medicine from the wall where it had been hanging and hand it back to the state. Salt Lake City had been this chelating physician's home since boyhood. He loved its surrounding mountains and forests. When Mormon patriarch Brigham Young looked upon the valley that comprises Salt Lake City today, he said, "This is the place!" It was the place for Dr. Vance and his family as well, but it isn't anymore.

USE OF THE MEDIA BY CHELATION THERAPY COMPETITION

Elmer R. Kanary of Massillon, Ohio, a patient desiring an opinion about chelation therapy from the American Medical Association (AMA), received a response from Asher J. Finkel, M.D., group vice president of the AMA's Divisions of Scientific Activities and Continuing Medical Studies, dated February 23, 1979: "We have always maintained that any licensed physician is free to use any drug that is approved by the Food and Drug Administration for marketing in any way that the physician deems it appropriate in his best clinical judgment. We have stated that the use of a drug is not restricted to the labeling that the FDA insists be attached to the drug or to advertising for that drug. Consequently, if your physician believes in the usefulness of chelation therapy for whatever purpose in his best clinical judgment, he is perfectly free to use it." Thus, the official policy of the AMA is that a physician is free to employ EDTA chelation therapy whenever he deems that it is in the best interest of the patient to do so!

Even so, it is not uncommon for national broadcasting media to follow the medical party line and present uninvestigated misinformation or erroneous old information on chelation therapy to the trusting public. Their most common pitch to prove the illegitimacy of chelation treatment is to say it's not accepted by the AMA, an untruthful statement as indicated by Dr. Finkel's letter. Or, the media may spout another irrelevancy that chelation therapy is a procedure for hardening of the arteries unapproved by the FDA.

The FDA has absolutely no jurisdiction over a medical doctor's practice. This agency only controls the marketing of drugs and medical devices across state lines for resale. In the sense that a pharmaceutical company or a manufacturer delivers its product and markets it in interstate commerce, the FDA can regulate what claims are made in its advertising and promotion. A physician is free to compound whatever medicines in his own expert and scientific opinion should be prescribed in the best interests of his patients. For a doctor to purchase ingredients and compound them into a prescription medicine in his office for his patients is not the marketing of a drug across state lines. And to even imply so is a far stretch of the imagination.

When the media declare to viewers or listeners that the FDA does not approve of a medicine's use for a physician-prescribed purpose, the media imply that the federal government somehow has authority to tell doctors how to practice medicine. This is not the truth at all. The FDA has no mandate to regulate physicians who use drugs and medical devices delivered in interstate commerce. That an FDA bureaucrat may feel differently tells us in some small measure on what kind of power trip some bureaucrats travel.

Certain national electronic media tend to disregard regulatory law this way. On the other hand, what may be worse is that the media people might not know the law as it relates to prescribing drugs, therapies, and medical practice. Possibly they just act out of ignorance of the facts. The Cable Health Network through reporting by Art Uhlene, M.D., in January 1983, communicated incorrect and outdated evidence on the efficacy and dangers of chelation therapy. I know because Dr. Uhlene's misstatements were thrown at me on the five o'clock news with Bob Donaldson as host, on KFDM-TV, in Beaumont, Texas. I was forced to take apart those wrong assertions and point out the falsehoods. And I previously described how the Turner Broadcasting System Inc., by means of its Cable News Network, in April 1983, did a hatchet job on H. Ray Evers, M.D., of Cottonwood, Alabama. I was in the Evers Health Center at the time doing two things: investigating Dr. Evers' treatment program for the book I am writing on *The Evers Odyssey* (no publisher yet) and taking chelation therapy myself. The Cable News Network reporters interviewed me but never broadcast any positive aspects of chelation therapy.

Then there is the vindictiveness of local doctors who are selling competitive treatment to patients. They easily fall into a routine of unfair competition by slandering chelation therapy. As in the Salt Lake City case, local city and town physicians practicing in the traditional mode habitually set naive media people to persecute a neighboring physician who provides intravenous infusions with EDTA. An incident happened in the Hartford, Connecticut, metropolitan area September 7, 8, and 9, 1983. Those were the three days that Hartford Station WFSB-TV, Channel 3, exhibited to viewers a number of fabrications and half-truths about chelation therapy. The TV reporter, Mary Ally Newman, provided just enough material to make it look really bad for Robert Harris, M.D., of Stafford Springs, Connecticut. Dr. Harris is the chelating physician whom Ms. Newman placed on the hot seat.

The three days of programming had the semblance of a conspiracy arrangement among at least three parties: WFSB-TV, FDA official Bruce Brown, and the president of the Hartford County Medical Society, Morris Seide, M.D., who practices in Hartford.

On the program, Dr. Seide testified against Dr. Harris. Knowing in advance that he was going to do this in his capacity as medical society president, Dr. Seide apologized to a mutual patient, a union president whom he also cared for independently of Dr. Harris. Under Dr. Harris's chelation therapy administrations, the patient was dramatically improving in his impaired peripheral vascular condition. Dr. Seide, the man's regular internist, was monitoring the condition's improvement and was favorably impressed with the results being observed in the patient from his chelation therapy. The patient, a member of the electrical contractor's union in Hartford, also expressed happiness at receiving 80 percent reimbursement of all of the health care costs associated with EDTA infusions. Dr. Seide was forced to agree with his patient that chelation therapy was doing a good job, but this did not stop the medical society president from going on television to publicly criticize both the treatment and the doctor administering it. The whole situation involved the usual medical politics. Besides Dr. Harris being a fall guy, the Hartford County viewers who suffer with cardiovascular diseases also became victims of this political game.

The Food and Drug Administration spokesman, Bruce Brown, was apparently involved with sending "bugged" patients to Dr. Harris. They had secretly been wired for recording their private conversations. These conversations were used as the basis for the television broadcasts.

Amazingly, Brown was critical of Dr. Harris's practice methods on the air and especially focused on the fact that the chelator dispensed books (which I had written) to patients that fully revealed all information about chelation therapy. Reading Chapter Six of *The Chelation Answer* provided the patient with full disclosure of "The Costs and Safety of Chelation Therapy," including technique of application, possible nephrotoxicity, any side effects, contraindications, drug incompatibilities, and interactions with EDTA. The patient who possessed this information was then able to give Dr. Harris informed consent to administer the treatment. Yet, Brown said that such books were a form of "labelling" at the point of sale of services.

Brown's implication was that the FDA somehow has authority to tell physicians how to practice medicine when this is not at all the case. It is forbidden by rulings against the FDA by the U.S. Supreme Court. And to advise that selling or giving away books is somehow a violation of the law borders strongly on constitutional infringement. Brown is obviously using his bureaucratic muscle to attempt to violate Dr. Harris's rights under the first amendment of the U.S. Constitution, or perhaps several other constitutional rights, including freedom of speech. He had given line by line critical commentary on the covertly recorded statements and Dr. Harris's responses about chelation therapy.

It also seems ludicrous that the FDA official, who claims that chelation therapy does not work, would in the next breath say "but it's going to loosen plaque and the plaque will lodge someplace else, causing serious problems." If he is going to claim it does not work, he cannot state that it is going to loosen plaque. And if he asserts that the plaque comes off the arterial walls, then chelation therapy must really be taking out the plaque and softening hardened arteries. Out of fairness to opponent arguments, I have to advise that it's possible that neither happens. Possibly, chelation treatment interrupts a disease process that allows plaque to heal gradually through normal body processes.

As for Dr. Morris Seide's criticism, he falls into the typical category of almost all doctor opponents of chelation therapy. Most of the physician enemies of this treatment have failed to use it, have no personal knowledge of it, and have no credentials to make them expert in any sort of opinion about chelation therapy. I challenge WFSB-TV to locate one physician anywhere in the country who has used EDTA intravenously on more than a dozen patients to reverse their atherosclerosis and who is not an advocate of this treatment. To my knowledge, all doctors having had any type of extensive experience in using chelation therapy to treat heart and artery diseases become strong proponents. The physicians who remain critics have no personal knowledge of chelation therapy whatsoever.

THE ASSOCIATION FOR CARDIOVASCULAR THERAPIES (ACT)

Chelation therapy and Dr. Robert Harris have their defenders. Among them is Audrey Goldman, executive director of the Association for Cardiovascular Therapies. Audrey went on WFSB-TV in response to the station's editorial. She asked if the government would sponsor medical research to see if chelation therapy is effective. One of the major problems with the treatment is that there is no source of funding. The FDA and the university cardiologists appearing on the program suggested that because no one had ever applied for an investigational new drug (IND) number, this somehow reflected badly on the treatment. This is not the case at all. There is absolutely no incentive for anyone to apply for an IND because of the inordinate amount of paperwork involved, the years of research needed (about eight), and the high cost of conducting the types of large-scale double-blind studies required by the Food and Drug Administration (approximately $30 million!) in order to include the indication of heart and artery diseases on the package insert.

WFSB-TV correctly stated that it is perfectly legal for a physician to use a drug approved by the FDA for one purpose and to adapt it for any other purpose that in the doctor's medical opinion is in the best interests of the patient. Thus there is no need to apply for an IND.

A drug company would certainly not apply for an IND, because the patent has long ago expired. There is no way any pharmaceutical manufacturer could protect its investment and recoup the research funds. It remains only for the federal government or some large philanthropy to do so, and from such institutions is where research money should come. With chelation therapy, it either works, and everyone should recognize it, or a very large-scale consumer fraud is taking place and the government should expose it.

But such investigations must be conducted scientifically, and not bombast the treatment with the slander and innuendo that is now the case.

The Association for Cardiovascular Therapies Inc. (ACT) does much more than respond to television editorials on chelation therapy. Founded in 1978, ACT is a national, non-profit holistic health organization, consisting of lay members and volunteers, many of them heart patients who have been helped by the ACT program. The organization has almost 100 chapters in operation across the United States. One of its important functions is the education and referral service for individuals seeking alternative therapies in the prevention and treatment of cardiovascular disease. ACT's staff responds to the many calls for help from families and patients suffering from a wide variety of degenerative diseases, such as heart disease, arthritis, stroke, senility, diabetes, and emphysema. The staff makes its response with great concern for extending life as well as relieving unnecessary pain and suffering, through the medical programs that ACT encourages.

ACT promptly answers phone calls and letters, and upon request packets of educational literature and doctor referral lists are mailed all over the country for only five dollars (for postage, printing, and handling). Literature is continually updated to bring the public the latest developments in the cardiovascular field. A wide variety of books and tapes are also available.

The goals of ACT include the following:

- To educate the public to the risk leading to cardiovascular disease and methods to prevent or minimize them.
- To seek fair treatment from health insurance companies and other third-party carriers such as the Department of Veterans Affairs. ACT is desirous of having alternative medical therapies paid for as readily as bypass surgery.
- To preserve and protect the patient-physician relationship in determining the method of treatment best suited for each patient against governmental or other outside intervention.
- To provide information on legislative, regulatory, and legal areas relating to cardiovascular health care coverage by Medicare and Medicaid.
- To inform the public of the most effective therapies at the most

reasonable cost for the prevention and treatment of cardiovascular disease.

- To broaden the narrow thinking of those who contribute to the current failures and inadequacies in the present treatment and prevention of the degenerative diseases of Western civilization.
- To raise funds for cardiovascular research.
- To establish ACT chapters in every major city in the United States.
- To prompt further research of drugs that no longer are protected by patent and, therefore, provide no incentive for pharmaceutical companies to invest in for further research or promotion.
- To offer medical training in chelation therapy to physicians, through ACT chapters.

Regular membership in ACT costs $25 per year.

Special membership costs $35 per year and a free book is included such as the hardcover *Chelation Therapy: How to Prevent or Reverse Hardening of the Arteries* by Dr. Morton Walker, the trade paperback of this book, *The Chelation Way: The Complete Book of Chelation Therapy,* or the booklet *The Healing Powers of Chelation Therapy* by John Parks Trowbridge, M.D., and Morton Walker, D.P.M.

You may reach the Association for Cardiovascular Therapies Inc. at its headquarters, 140 Huyshope Ave., Hartford, Connecticut 06106; (203) 724-0081.

THE HEALTH HISTORY OF JOHN SORENSON

John Sorenson of Oklahoma City, a retired U.S. Air Force Colonel, is awed by what chelation therapy has done in restoring his own life. John Sorenson tells his health history and highly dramatic story:

"For as far back as I can remember, I have had a grossly insufficient memory and an inadequate ability to select the really important facts from the tons of ideas we meet and deal with each day," wrote John Sorenson in a case history that he furnished for publication. "I could never outline a study lesson and couldn't remember classroom lectures. I had to study four times as hard as other kids just to barely pass school courses. Although I was able to put together a fairly successful career and life, the fact remains that, without these learning disabilities, I could have achieved at least a 25 percent more successful life than I did. This is important for you to know, as the end of this case history will show.

"Starting with high blood pressure, in 1974, my health began to decline. A doctor put me on medication and said that I would have to take blood pressure medicines the rest of my life. Next came headaches, then insomnia, obesity, lack of vigor, alternating halo and center-of-field-of-vision blind spots. I had a hypersensitivity of vision and skin to sunlight, developed psoriasis and skin lesions on the forehead. Skin sloughed off of my finger tips and elbows; hay fever symptoms became more pronounced and my feet, ankles, knees, and shoulders began to hurt most of the time. My temper would flare for no apparent reason." Sorenson admits that he was a wreck.

"In 1977, the doctors discovered that I had developed heart arrhythmia [an irregular heartbeat]. I had been running a flight training and aircraft rental operation following my retirement from the Air Force, but I had to quit this job because I found myself unable to pass the physical and functional qualifications of a commercial pilot. The doctors prescribed Inderal™, Quinidine™, Esidrix™, and Klorvess™ for helping my heart problem. My memory became even worse as did my ability to evaluate and reason."

With the passage of time Sorenson anticipated his own early death. He writes: "By 1981, I had lost all hope of surviving for very much longer. I knew that I was dying but there wasn't a thing I could do about it.

"Impotence set in. I know of nothing that will kill a man's self-respect as efficiently as having difficulty with getting an erection. My vigor practically disappeared, and then I was struck with anginal chest pains. There were many weeks that I spent doing nothing but sitting back all day in my Lazy Boy rocker. I accepted my death and made plans to go out as gracefully as possible with a minimum of inconvenience to loved ones." Sorenson had given up entirely.

"About this time a very dear friend had sustained a heart attack. Tests, including an angiogram, indicated that he had a high percentage of arterial blockage in five different locations on and around his heart. The tests also showed that he could not tolerate bypass surgery. The doctors told him to go home, get his affairs in order and take pain killers to make his demise more comfortable. But another of our friends told him about chelation therapy. He tried it and the supportive therapies of the holistic treatment regimen, including oral chelating agents and exercise. His recovery was miraculous.

"My loving wife saw this and began a campaign to get me to go and try chelation therapy too," Sorenson says. "Finally, in January 1982 I was persuaded to go to the Genesis Medical Center in Oklahoma City, Oklahoma. The staff gave me a seven-page questionnaire to fill out and an appointment to see the center's director, Charles Farr, M.D., Ph.D., a week later. The health history questionnaire was so detailed and searching that I had to really work to complete it.

"At that visit with Dr. Farr, I found him friendly, self-assured, business-like, and I immediately liked the man. He told me that he practiced holistic medicine, including the use of natural food eating, vitamins, minerals, exercise, stress control, and an absolute minimum of patent or prescription medicines. This is paradoxical when you consider that Dr. Farr's Ph.D. is in pharmacology. He explained that we each live in a chemical factory, that when its chemical balances are disrupted illness happens, that he could test me and determine what was right, what was wrong, and what to do to correct deficiencies. He recommended 12 tests for me to take, and I agreed. Dr. Farr handed me three half-gallon plastic jugs for urine samples, and I told him if he wanted them filled that day we both were in big trouble," Sorenson writes.

"The holistic physician explained that I was to fast for 24 hours the following day and fill the first bottle. For the second day I was to eat as always and fill the second bottle. Then I was to fast on the third day and fill bottle number three. In this way he could evaluate my renal (kidney) function over a 72-hour period rather than the standard 70 minutes from the usual five-ounce sample. Among my other tests the staff checked blood pressure in both of my arms, both of my legs, all my fingers and toes. They tested volumetric blood flow, the digestive system, heart function during stress, and a host of other things.

"Two weeks later I met with Dr. Farr again for about 45 minutes. He held a copy of my test results, handed me a copy to keep, turned on a tape recorder, and we reviewed the information the papers contained. Our words were tape recorded, and the physician gave me the tape which I have used many times to review my medical history," said Sorenson.

"I was stunned when Dr. Farr asked if I knew that I was in chronic kidney failure. He said that I was allergic to nine of the foods I had been eating regularly, and they had been poisoning my system, probably all my life. The doctor placed me on an anti-allergy rotation diet engineered for me personally, a regimen of vitamins and minerals specifically chosen for my needs, a stress control program tailored for counteracting what had been pulling me down, plus exercise and attitude enforcement programs designed for me personally.

"In two months I had lost 25 pounds, had loads of vigor, was walking rapidly four miles per day, slept like a baby, and was rapidly regaining my health, feeling better than ever before," explained Sorenson. "During this time I had counted up all of the symptoms of ill health I had started with and came up with 66 symptoms. By the end of the third month over half of them had been reversed. I was meeting other patients who were undergoing chelation therapy and each told me how their poor circulation and related problems were being overcome by these treatments.

"I asked Dr. Farr to give me chelation therapy and, since he believed it would provide me with benefits, I took 20 intravenous infusions a week apart. During the nineteenth treatment I mentioned that I could detect no particular improvements in my blood flow, and then my wife advised me that my hair, which had been falling out at a rapid rate, was now growing back.

"Two weeks later some friends had invited us to Little Rock, Arkansas, to see their new home. My wife wrote down instructions, containing seven changes, to get to the house. As we left Oklahoma City my wife read the directions to me," said Sorenson. "When we reached Little Rock I repeated the instructions back almost verbatim. Remember what I said in the first paragraph about having such a poor memory? For 67 years my life had been seriously impaired by a totally inadequate ability to remember things. I had faulty reasoning power. Do you have a child who isn't able to learn? Have his teachers assured you that the child is just lazy as happened in my case? All this time it possibly was poor circulation or food allergy for me. Might that be your child's problem?

"Since taking chelation therapy my life has been a constant process of improving health, happiness, and productivity," continued Sorenson. "But I have one small problem. I'm having to learn how to be a totally new me, a person with a normal memory and reasoning power. Needless to say, I am happy with this new me, and the expanded self-assurance I have acquired. And I am taking one chelation booster treatment each month as a prevention method against further illness. I want no return to the health unhappiness I lived with all my life. No child should ever be subjected to such an unhappy existence.

"The following is a list of major benefits chelation therapy has provided me: improved hair growth, freedom from headaches, a good memory, ability to think clearly, no aches and pains except from physical injuries, clear vision, the ability to walk up to eight miles a day, weight loss to a normal 175 pounds, reversal of impotency, a healthy, tough, and flexible skin, a better skin color, bright, red blood color versus muddy looking blood, no skin eruptions, wounds that heal twice as quickly as before, and no hyperacidity. I have won back 25 years of my life. At age 68, I am doing more and better work than I did at age 40," writes John Sorenson. "I declare this honestly and will repeat it on the telephone to anyone who calls me at home at (405) 721-3329, or who writes to me at my residence, 8016 West Lakeshore Drive, Oklahoma City, Oklahoma 73132."

CHAPTER EIGHT

The Current Status of Chelation Therapy

EDTA chelation therapy pioneer E. W. McDonagh, D.O., and the other staff members at the McDonagh Medical Center in Kansas City, Missouri, launched and then dropped a lawsuit on behalf of all patients across the country against major health insurance companies who have failed to reimburse their policy holders for chelation treatments. Dr. McDonagh, backed by his clinical administrator, William D. Johnson, and his chief counsel, Joe Teasdale, who is the former governor of Missouri, filed the case March 30, 1983, as an anti-trust action against national Blue Cross, national Blue Shield, Travelers Insurance Company, Prudential Insurance Company, plus five county medical societies from the Kansas City area. Other chelating physicians and their patients were adding support.

The suit charged "unlawful combination and conspiracy" between insurance companies and medical societies to restrain trade in denying coverage for chelation treatments. The insurers and associated medical societies were also charged with engaging in a restraint of interstate trade and commerce in the nonpayment of health and medical services rendered by chelation doctors to patients insured by the defendant insurance companies. Attorney Richard Knight, a law associate of Joe Teasdale, said plaintiff attorneys, before the case was dropped, were in the process of conducting discovery and filing motions to prevent some of the defendants from obtaining removal from the suit. A decision was made in early

1985 neither to proceed as individual plaintiffs suing the individual defendants nor as a class action.

The case would have cost Dr. McDonagh and his voluntary contributors (mostly chelating physicians) at least $400,000 in legal fees, and so it was dropped.

A victory for plaintiffs would have set a landmark precedent compelling insurers to reimburse for chelation therapy and other alternative therapies. It was being led by a dynamic attorney. Former Governor Teasdale is a long-time foe of the insurance industry in Missouri. During his term as governor from 1977 to 1981, he had been involved in preventing insurance companies from exploiting the people. Also, Joe Teasdale, before and since his governorship, has participated in numerous litigations encompassing such insurance enterprises.

Why might chelation therapists have taken this unprecedented action? Because medical insurance companies, including Medicare, have traditionally paid for very expensive surgical procedures such as the coronary artery bypass operation without question. They have made these payments even in the face of having no controlled double-blind studies to prove safety and effectiveness. Yet, this is the criteria—double-blind studies—demanded of chelation therapy to have it reimbursed by health insurers.

Too often patients like Harold Pryor of Cleveland, Ohio, whom I report on in the next section, are not covered for undertaking a life-saving treatment such as chelation therapy. Instead, they are forced into accepting surgery or other procedures that put their lives in danger. It's a case of being able to pay for the surgical care and not the chelation care. Oftentimes the patients will get all of their medical costs covered by health insurance if policy holders submit their bodies to open heart surgery, leg artery bypass, cardiac sympathectomy, leg amputation, or some other dangerous operation generally recognized by health insurance carriers.

An assumption has been made right along that angiographic evidence of occlusion with follow-up evidence of improved blood flow was sufficient justification for surgery. A chelating physician in Cleveland, James P. Frackelton, M.D., former president of the ACAM, co-authored with Elmer Cranton, M.D., an important article on the "Current Status of EDTA Chelation Therapy in Occlusive Arterial Disease" (published in the *Journal of Holistic Medicine*,

Volume 4, Number 1, Spring/Summer 1982, pages 24-33). The two authors wrote: "It has never been demonstrated that this [improved blood flow] is the major or only reason for relief of symptoms. A number of years ago cardiac sympathectomy was used to effectively relieve angina. Perhaps cardiac sympathectomy (cutting of nerves in the heart muscle), which inevitably accompanies coronary artery bypass surgery, results in subsequent improvement of blood vessel spasm and is more important than other factors in post-surgical improvement of angina."

MEDICARE GIVES HAROLD PRYOR HIS "FAIR HEARING"

If you submit your health insurance claim for reimbursement from an insurance carrier in your area representing Medicare and that claim is denied, you are entitled to what the Social Security Administration calls "a fair hearing." When it comes to adjudicating reimbursement to you for chelation therapy, it's seldom fair.

Harold Pryor had been under the care of Dr. James Frackleton for chelation therapy for extensive occlusive vascular disease, involving the coronary arteries, the cerebral arteries, and the arteries in his extremities. They were functioning only minimally. The treatment was "reasonable and necessary," a couple of favorite terms bandied about by health insurers. Mr. Pryor had experienced frequent episodes of transient blindness, lasting up to a week at a time. He also had other symptoms of transient ischemic attack, suggesting that he suffered with ulcerating plaque in his carotid arteries.

Pryor's previous doctors had recommended that he go for diagnostic angiograms, with probable carotid artery surgery and/or coronary artery bypass surgery coming down as the final verdict. Pryor believed that he would not survive such operations. Having sustained six heart attacks already, the patient had significant coronary artery occlusive disease and was legally determined, since 1956, to be entirely disabled by the state of Ohio because of arteriosclerotic heart disease. The patient elected instead to take his chelation therapy series of injections in 1980 and promptly filed a Medicare claim for reimbursement. Just as promptly he was denied payment, Medicare declaring that the "investigational" treatment was "unreasonable and unnecessary." Further pursuit of the claim by his request for a fair hearing did get him a small reimbursement for his thermographic studies.

A year later, the patient again took a series of chelation treatments, including thermographic studies to check on his progress. This time Medicare's local health insurance carrier representative, Nationwide Mutual Insurance Company, refused not only reimbursement of the EDTA infusions but also denied payment for the thermography. The previous year's favorable ruling during the fair hearing carried no weight for thermographic reimbursement the next time. So, Pryor again requested a fair hearing.

This second time, at two separate hearings held in April and May 1981, Pryor's chelating physician, Dr. James Frackelton, attended in order to give testimony and personally paid travel costs for the board chairman of the ACAM, Garry F. Gordon, M.D., from North Highlands, California, as an expert witness to support the patient's claim. Dr. Gordon gave of his time at no charge.

The "fair hearing" officer, Max. J. Clark, Esq., seemed rather upset when the extra chelation physician appeared at the appointed location, a room in the Holiday Inn in Middleburgh Heights, Ohio, with the patient and his wife. A Medicare patient requesting a fair hearing is entitled to bring anyone as his witness. Not only had Mr. and Mrs. Pryor been accompanied by a high powered expert, but also Dr. Frackelton had arranged to have along their own court reporter, three tape recorders, and Mrs. Marilyn Frackelton, as general assistant to the distressed elderly couple.

"Fair hearing" officer Clark failed to provide enough time for Pryor's presentation. Although the patient's appointment began at 2:00 p.m., the government man had scheduled another hearing at 3:30 p.m. Pryor's testimony on the advanced state of his prior condition (to make it clear that his chelation treatment was "reasonable and necessary"), his wife's corroboration regarding the extent of his illness, copies of his previous medical records, Dr. Frackelton's testimony, and a local attorney's testimony all had to be presented at the next hearing, over a month later. The medical expert on chelation therapy testified at the first part of the hearing inasmuch as he had traveled thousands of miles to aid Pryor's case and wasn't about to make a second trip.

During the course of the presentations, Max Clark admitted on the record that he was biased against chelation treatment. He said that he had been the officer in charge of at least four previous chelation therapy hearings and had always routinely denied all reimbursement. But, said the government employee, this time he would "make an independent decision today," relating to the facts, and not based on any other opinions. He lied! The "fair hearing" officer came back ten months later and said, "I reviewed the matter with medical consultants. As a result of this evaluation, I have determined the use of EDTA for Mr. Pryor's medical condition is still investigational and cannot be considered reasonable or necessary." Harold Pryor collected nothing from Medicare. It didn't matter to the patient anymore. Clark had delayed his decision until a month after the retiree had died.

The patient had required more chelation therapy and could not afford it. The Pryors had used up their life savings, which had originally been put away for use in retirement. Medicare figuratively just shrugged its bureaucratic shoulders. It implied by its rulings that it was willing to let the patient undergo open heart surgery or have him get his carotid arteries mechanically cleaned out. For this the agency would pay medical costs, but it refused to pay for the safer technique of chemical endarterectomy.

The inevitable happened! Despite the fact that Harold Pryor had experienced a remarkable turnaround with his health and returned to performing heavier work at home, discontinuing his chelation therapy took its toll. You could probably say, in effect, that the decision arrived at by Medicare had killed the man.

WHY ESTABLISHMENT MEDICINE OPPOSES
CHELATION THERAPY

Almost all of the opposition to chelation therapy by establishment medicine derives mainly from one published report in the scientific literature that attempts to disprove the effectiveness of intravenous EDTA therapy. A 1963 medical journal article by J.R. Kitchell, M.D., F. Palmon, M.D., N. Aytan, M.D., and L. E. Meltzer, M.D., "The Treatment of Coronary Artery Disease With Disodium EDTA, A Reappraisal," published in the *American Journal of Cardiology* 11:501-506, is the culprit. Reappraising their own positive studies of 1960 with subsequent additional patients, they repeatedly cite disapproval of the effectiveness of EDTA therapy. But the authors are wrong in their conclusion, something discernible to most scientists reading the full article. When you read the authors' summary, it is contrary to their data. The majority of patients in that "reappraisal" were reported to have improved and to have maintained improvement following their infusion with the ethylene diamine tetraacetic acid.

Moreover, Drs. Cranton and Frackelton, in their article that I have cited earlier, point out: "After 18 months with no further therapy and with no stated dietary or risk factor modification, 46 percent of a group of 28 patients remained improved. Twenty-three of those 28 patients had suffered previous myocardial infarctions. The conclusion in that paper that EDTA therapy was not effective, because some patients regressed when treatment was discontinued, is not justified. There is no other treatment about which the same sort of statement could not be made, including coronary artery bypass surgery."

In order to assess this 1963 "reappraisal" that has created this vast amount of trouble between medical traditionalists and chelation therapists, check out the twenty-eight patients. What happened to them after they received twenty chelation treatments? More than 64 percent were rated as improved; 71 percent had subjective improvement of symptoms; 64 percent had objective improvement of measured exercise tolerance three months later; and 46 percent showed improved electrocardiographic patterns. At the end of eighteen months, 46 percent remained improved. These results are very impressive and unquestionably do not support the authors' negative evaluation.

In retrospect, it's the article's conclusion that most physicians read when investigating the efficacy of chelation therapy. It appears that the authors' summary in that "reappraisal" article is, to a great extent, responsible for lack of subsequent funding for chelation therapy research, the cessation of clinical trials with EDTA, the wide rift between exponents and opponents of the therapy, refusal of cost reimbursement by insurance companies, harassment of chelating physicians by orthodox medical societies, and much more difficulty. Yet, this "reappraisal" article is just one negative report out of approximately 2,000 other positive ones published in the medical literature. Still, it's the only one that is pointed at by medical orthodoxy to support its anti-chelation therapy arguments.

Then, critics of EDTA infusions point to a brief review article by P. C. Craven, M.D., and H. F. Morrelli, M.D., ("Chelation Therapy." *Western Journal of Medicine* 122:277-278, 1975), which is based on obsolete studies written by scientists with no personal expertise in the use of EDTA injections for occlusive arterial disease. Craven and Morrelli state in their conclusion that because funds have not been provided for large-scale, multi-variant, double-blind controlled studies that would satisfy the FDA's requirement for inclusion of occlusive arterial disease on the package insert, the use of EDTA should be " . . . conducted under carefully controlled conditions in an academic institution by experienced investigators." Such a statement insults the clinical competence and judgment of those many experienced physicians in private practice who have been safely using intravenous EDTA for decades.

ASSESSING THE SAFETY OF CHELATION THERAPY

EDTA chelation therapy has been accused of being toxic to the kidneys. In fact, rather than being nephrotoxic, the treatment can actually be beneficial to the kidneys. Adults with chronic lead exposure show interstitial nephritis and high blood pressure. Physicians using chelation therapy for them frequently see improved kidney function reflected by improved creatinine clearance and reduction of the elevated blood pressure. I pointed this out in Chapter Five when citing some of the McDonagh, Rudolph, Cheraskin reports. Opponents who point to nephrotoxicity have never read the latest published papers.

When television commentators or media-guest doctors say that chelation therapy can be dangerous, of course, the statement is correct. That's why EDTA is a prescription drug. Possible hazard is the reason it must be administered by a physician who is fully trained and has a solid scientific background. Most prescription drugs are dangerous. It's just a question of how dangerous they are and which is the greater risk—the disease being treated or the drug being prescribed.

To put this in perspective, the number of patients receiving chelation therapy is approximately half the number of those receiving coronary artery bypass surgery. Maybe two million patients have received coronary artery bypass operations (over 250,000 in the last year). Using a conservative average estimate, of the patients who have received bypass surgery, 3 percent have died either during or shortly after surgery as a direct result of the operation. This means that approximately 60,000 people have died under the surgeon's knife. And this does not even address the much greater numbers who have suffered long-term complications of pain, invalidism, disability, constant drug taking, and more. The complications from surgery were not severe enough to result in immediate death, but suffering with complications became a living death for heart surgery's victims.

Now look at the number of people who have undergone chelation therapy. In its vendetta against doctors giving EDTA infusions, the FDA has been able to search out only ten cases of death at the most in the past thirty years possibly traceable to chelation treatment. This means that the danger of death from bypass surgery is about 6,000 times greater than for chelation therapy.

If you give table salt in too large a quantity, too rapidly, you can kill a person. Is table salt dangerous? Each year 50,000 Americans die in auto accidents. Do we avoid riding in automobiles because of this reason? Danger is entirely relative.

Certainly EDTA is potentially toxic to the kidneys if it is not administered properly. Dr. Elmer Cranton, who is a past president of the American Holistic Medical Association, formerly second vice president of the American College of Advancement in Medicine, diplomate in the American Board of Family Practice, says as a rebuttal to media critics of chelation therapy such as the Hartford, Connecticut, television station WFSB, whose anti-chelation program I had discussed in Chapter Seven: "I think that to try to defend physicians who do not do thorough prechelation evaluations and who do not follow their patients kidney functions and other problems adequately should not be defended by us [ACAM]. I think that it is analogous to stating that because one surgeon happens to be a bungler and 30 percent of his patients undergoing gallbladder surgery die, therefore, gallbladder surgery is a dangerous and bad form of treatment. You should look to the experts in surgery before forming a conclusion rather than picking out the least skillful." The same holds true for chelation therapy.

Dr. Cranton went on to say that a physician who has gone before the American Board of Chelation Therapy and passed its requirements, demonstrating competence, can be relied upon. "If the therapy is being administered by physicians who do not conduct thorough pre-treatment physical examinations, with proper medical testing, and who do not test the kidney functions with each infusion, they are not doing this chelation therapy according to the approved and accepted safe methods, and should be shunned. Physicians who do not totally inform their patients of the treatment's bad press, who do not tell their patients about everything that could possibly go wrong, who do not advise their patients of all the alternatives available to them, who do not inform their patients that, indeed, there is a small but measurable risk of kidney failure, ending in renal dialysis for life, deserve entirely what comes to them," Dr. Cranton said.

"Physicians who imply that everyone will improve with chelation therapy, who assure that this is a treatment giving 100 percent results, or who guarantee results, deserve everything they get. With friends like those, the chelation therapy movement does not need enemies. So certainly," concluded Dr. Cranton, "what the treatment's enemies are saying about chelation can be stated about any prescription medicine used many times every day by just about every doctor. It is dangerous, and it is unproved. But these same statements could also be said of the vast majority of treatments used by physicians around the world daily in their practices."

ASSESSING THE EFFICACY OF MEDICAL TECHNOLOGIES

In 1978, Congress commissioned the Office of Technology Assessment (OTA) to investigate and issue a report on "Assessing the Efficacy and Safety of Medical Technologies" in the United States (for sale by the Superintendent of Documents, U.S. Government Printing Office, Washington, D.C. 20402, Stock Number 052-003-00593-0). In this study it states that only 10 to 20 percent of all procedures used in present medical practice have been shown to be of benefit by controlled clinical trials. It clearly says that many of the procedures (the other 80 to 90 percent) may not be effective. The assessors talk at length about coronary artery bypass surgery. Do you realize that over 210,000 such operations were carried out in 1988 at an average cost of $60,000 for surgeon and hospital? This means the one operation, coronary artery bypass, brings orthodox medicine more than $12 billion a year. It's a major industry in itself. Chelation therapy costs less than a tenth that of bypass surgery. Here is what the OTA report states about coronary bypass:

> Approximately 25,000 operations were performed in 1973 and at least 70,000 in 1977. Yet the benefits of coronary bypass surgery have not been clearly demonstrated. Claims that the operation prevents death remain largely unproven . . . The hospital mortality rate for patients undergoing such surgery is reported between 0.3 and 8 percent, with a usual range of 1 to 4 percent. However, only good results are published, generally, and the operative mortality rate derived from a large number of hospitals providing comparable data was 4 percent in 1976. Some other complications include myocardial infarction during surgery, in about 7 percent of patients.

In another location the OTA report says that of those therapies that were presumed to have been proven effective by studies, nearly 75 percent of scientific papers analyzed would have to be declared invalid or insupportable in their conclusions as a result of statistical problems alone. Also blamed for incorrect therapeutic assessment were poor research design, data collection errors, and analysis of specific areas of medicine relating to those studied.

The Office of Technology Assessment (OTA) wrote nothing about chelation therapy. But I suggest that it could be dangerous, and this statement is true of almost everything else physicians use in the practice of medicine. Otherwise, a prescription would not be required and people would be able to buy any medicine or medical device without a prescription. It's just a question of the relative risk, minimizing the risk by expert use, and the physician providing for the patient that service which he believes to be in the best interest of the patient.

IN THE BEST INTEREST OF JACKEE DAVIDSON

Ever since childhood, Jackee Davidson, formerly of Vernon, Connecticut, was considered hypochondriacal (excessively concerned about her health). Her pediatricians could find no particular cause, and Jackee's symptoms, more often than not, were dismissed as imaginary.

At the age of 29 Mrs. Davidson was on her own in a high-powered business and raising two children. Her symptoms continued. They consisted of heavy pressure behind the right eye causing it to feel as if the eyeball were being forced out of its socket, shortness of breath, headaches, chest pains, leg cramps, diarrhea, and nausea. She spent a great amount of time and money with doctors and hospitals. The medical professionals took all kinds of tests, including blood work, electroencephalograms, electrocardiograms, brain scans—you name it, and Jackee Davidson had experienced the diagnostic procedures. She was told, "You are in a high stress business. Don't worry, you'll live to be 100. Your problem is just 'nerves.' Try to relax more."

The symptoms were a constant daily source of agony for her, but she had learned to live with them. Upon questioning, Davidson told me, "I began to be afraid to go to a doctor. I didn't want to hear about my 'nerves' anymore. I tried to ignore the pain, hoping it would go away. Of course it didn't. And then the blockage occurred which nearly cost me my life. It wasn't just nerves after all."

The woman suffered a stroke. March 3, 1978, in the middle of the night, while she was living in Virginia Beach, Virginia, Davidson sustained a cerebral vascular accident after first feeling a series of familiar symptoms. She had vomiting, diarrhea, profuse sweating, dizziness, and joint pains. She thought she had contracted a virus flu. After taking some aspirin and going to bed, Davidson slept fitfully for about ninety minutes. It was then that she awakened to horrible excruciating pain radiating through her whole left side. Her body parts on the left side were paralyzed, swollen, and colored greyish purple.

Davidson's telephone was only two inches from her bed, but it took her forty-five minutes to reach the handpiece to call for help. One side of her mouth couldn't function. The friend that she finally reached called the emergency medical technician squad of Virginia Beach. They took her to Virginia Beach's Doctors Hospital where they refused her admission because of a lack of facilities. The squad then brought her to DePaul Hospital in Norfolk, where she remained. An angiogram of her blocked arteries was taken.

"Anyone who has had an angiogram knows what a horror it is," Davidson said. "I had three. Blockages were found in both legs, left shoulder, and in the aorta. I asked if there was any alternative to bypass surgery and was told 'no, there is absolutely nothing and if you want to live, we must operate quickly.' The vascular surgeon replaced the descending aorta and upper iliacs with a dacron graft."

While she was recuperating, the surgical team came in and told her that three more bypasses were required. "You have three more extensive blockages that need repair. We want you back here in two months for us to operate on both of your legs, then in four months we'll do more work on your arteries." When Davidson said that she did not intend to return for more surgery, the doctors replied, "Well you better be back because otherwise, you'll be dead in a year." Asking for any dietary restrictions or supplementary help she could give herself, the surgeons' only response was that she "stay away from too many fats and dairy products."

"Meantime, I had to put my life in order. The illness and lack of medical insurance had bankrupted me," admits Davidson. "I could not return to my profession, which had far too much physical as well as mental stress. I moved to Roanoke, Virginia, got a job as a receptionist, and spent every spare moment learning and studying at Unity of Roanoke Valley, whose Truth Principles teach a very positive, loving attitude and way of life. It was there, at a workshop about holistic medicine, that I heard answers to all of my questions the doctors in the hospital could not, or would not, answer. I began to pray for a way to be treated by the lecturer, Elmer M. Cranton, M.D., of Trout Dale, Virginia, so that I could live longer than just the one more year predicted. Time was running out, even though I was still a young woman.

"Six months later the graft in my right leg clogged and gangrene infected my foot. At the hospital, amputation of my leg was recommended. Then the miracle occurred. Friends from Unity of Roanoke Valley made arrangements for me to be treated at Dr. Cranton's clinic. They packed and moved me in a trailer that was parked on the clinic lot, with an intercom system hooked into where I had to lay," she explained.

The Cranton clinic in Trout Dale is located in a mountain setting. Dr. Cranton began chelation therapy the next day, trying to save the patient's leg. By trial and error, the chelating physician discovered that Davidson was extremely sensitive to EDTA and other ingredients in the intravenous solution. Repeatedly, he had to slow the drip, space the treatments farther apart, and cut the dosage. In fact, the first time she took the treatment, even following the ACAM protocol, his patient had a grand mal seizure (an epileptic convulsion of major proportions). To avoid any more sensitivity reactions, Dr. Cranton elected to slow down the treatment to the minimum level. About once a week, at 9:00 p.m., he would enter the trailer and hook the patient into the chelating solution IV, setting the solution speed to drip for twelve hours. He taught Davidson how to unhook herself at 9:00 a.m. the next morning. This was the only way she could take chelation therapy; otherwise, the woman would experience body cramps, joint pain, headache, nausea, and other side effects.

"Although it was many months before my foot healed and intermittent claudication disappeared, during this time I joyfully worked in the clinic, learned how to prepare and cook food for patients with degenerative diseases, counseled and inspired other chelation therapy patients, studied and became a certified emergency medical technician, and got to meet and care deeply for the wonderful, warm, loving mountain people," said Davidson. "The eighteen months I was privileged to spend at the clinic in southwest Virginia were the happiest, most productive, love-filled months of my life."

Jackee Davidson did not lose her right leg. She walks on it now and worked for a time in Bloomfield, Connecticut, at the Association for Cardiovascular Therapies Inc. (ACT), where she occasionally acted as a volunteer. Without any financial reward, she assisted people in need as she had been aided. Jackee is content that she may have helped other people the way that she was helped by the loving people of another holistic organization. Mrs. Davidson says, "The joy it is to work with such dedicated professionals and lay persons, and to be given the opportunity to help educate people who are seeking knowledge or preventive medicine, nutrition, chelation therapy, and the holistic approach was an answer to my prayers."

PART TWO
Oral Chelating Agents for Cardiovascular Self-Help at Home

CHAPTER NINE

The Concept of Oral Chelation Therapy

While attending a business conference in New York City, and with no prior warning that it was coming upon him, 48-year-old factory owner and industrial executive Jack Bodolay of Lakeland, Florida, was struck suddenly by a massive myocardial infarction. His heart attack was complicated by extremely high blood pressure that resisted correction by nearly all forms of anti-hypertensive medication, as well as sedatives.

Mr. Bodolay managed to survive the perilous episode and with the passage of time did return to very limited activity. His lifestyle altered. He was restricted in the amount of work he could do, and as a result of residual angina pectoris, the executive's physical movements were cut down to a minimum. His body's response to many forms of heart medicines and blood pressure drugs was poor. The medical advice given to him was to consider coronary artery bypass surgery for possibly reducing the angina.

A family member came to Bodolay one day with information about chelation therapy and the potential benefits experienced by other individuals with his same history and current physical condition. Being a studious and well-educated person, the industrial executive did a rather thorough and scholarly investigation on his own of this totally unfamiliar treatment. He checked into where chelation injections were administered in the Lakeland area, resulting in his calling for further firsthand information and answers to questions that Bodolay put to Robert J. Rogers, M.D., of Melbourne, Florida. Dr. Rogers is renowned in Florida as a chelating physician because he won a landmark decision at the Florida Supreme Court level against the Florida State Board of Medical Examiners in favor of chelation therapy and in favor of retaining his license to practice medicine. In their written decision, the Supreme Court justices compared Dr. Rogers to Pasteur, Copernicus, and Freud.

Not yet knowing of the Florida Supreme Court's judgment, Bodolay coincidentally went so far as to call the Florida State Board of Medical Examiners, although he guessed in advance that as representatives of organized medicine the board members would probably take a public stand in opposition to this non-traditional treatment. George Palmer, M.D., who at the time of the cardiac patient's phone call was executive director of the examining board, had only negative remarks to make about chelation therapy. He continued to speak in this critical way until the patient asked the $64 question.

"Doctor, please help me with this dilemma that I am in. Here is my situation," Jack Bodolay remembers saying, "I'm a relatively young man and love life and love my family. I have a large manufacturing company with its many responsibilities. I have investigated my options of [1] continuing therapy on the present drugs, without surgery (and I fear and dread the surgical possibilities) or [2] I could, in addition, go ahead with bypass surgery if I could overcome the fears I have of the significant mortality risks of the operation and the failures that I have learned about which all too often seem to result following the surgery. I'm miserable with the incomplete response I am making on all these drugs. Now, Dr. Palmer, off the record, if you were me, what would you do?"

The answer that came back to the patient was, "Since there is no evidence that what Rogers is doing seems to be harmful and feeling the way you say you do, I would go down to Melbourne and have Rogers give me chelation therapy. That's strictly off the record."

(Reader, since I am an investigative medical journalist and true names and statements are mandatory in my reporting, and since I made no promises to anyone to keep Dr. Palmer's beliefs off the record, you are reading them here.)

When Jack Bodolay had recovered from the shock of hearing the true thoughts of the executive director of the Florida State Board of

Medical Examiners, he thanked the doctor for his candid reply. This orthodox doctor's honesty probably contributed to extending the man's life. He was persuaded to undertake a series of chelation treatments.

More of my probing into the patient's medical history reveals that he had a surprisingly favorable outcome as a result of his treatment at the Rogers Clinic of Preventive Medicine. Bodolay's angina pain subsided after fifteen to twenty intravenous infusions with EDTA. His more recalcitrant elevated blood pressure did not come down to normal until the forty-fifth treatment. Since then, it has fluctuated in a normal range.

The man was a compliant patient who commuted regularly for his IV therapy by means of his corporate aircraft. But he also was faithful in the way he followed the lifestyle improvements that are a part of the overall chelation therapy program. He adapted well to a complete self-help procedure that he adjusted to wherever he happened to be—at home, at work, or at recreation. He became involved in a prudent graduated exercise program of walking and jogging. This form of self-chelation activity began following his twentieth IV treatment. He ate the chelating form of diet and markedly reduced or eliminated the drinking of alcoholic beverages that usually accompanies corporate life. More than that, Dr. Rogers had placed the patient on numerous nutritional supplements that tend to act as oral chelating agents. The nutrients also assisted Bodolay's body in correcting metabolic dysfunctions such as hypoglycemia and allergies as well as elevated readings of his blood cholesterol and triglycerides. High-density lipoprotein levels increased in his blood from taking the oral chelators. Moreover, being a world traveler and business executive, Bodolay was able to get some of the oral chelating medicinal substances that have been well proven to the food and drug administrations of foreign countries. Dr. Rogers agrees that in Europe and Japan these medications, while not as dramatically effective as IV chelation therapy, have been reported to lessen the progression of the thickening and plugging of the arteries. I report on such medicinal oral chelates in detail in Chapter Twelve.

With the overabundant psychological stress of his business stringently reduced, his much needed physical exercise assiduously increased, the high blood pressure lowered to normal, and the hardened arteries made to reverse the disease process, Bodolay's life is no longer threatened. Almost four years after his heart attack, the man enjoys a normal lifestyle from a physical activities' aspect. He jogs three miles around the lakeshore in his neighborhood. The only restriction that he has is to avoid those foods that caused his original problem. The man takes no heart stimulants or blood pressure drugs, remains on oral nutritional chelating agents for their maintenance value, and continues to receive booster treatments with intravenous EDTA at six-to-twelve-month intervals. Jack Bodolay considers all of his various lifestyle changes welcome in view of the other unpleasant alternatives he was offered before learning of intravenous and oral chelation therapy.

WHAT IS ORAL CHELATION THERAPY?

Biochemist Richard Passwater, Ph.D., of Berlin, Maryland, director of research for the Solgar Company Inc., has been credited with first using the term "oral chelation" when referring to specific foods and nutritional supplements that help to cleanse the blood vessels of accumulated detritus and improve blood flow. Robert Downs, D.C., clinic director of the Southwest Center of the Healing Arts in Albuquerque, New Mexico, acted on the concept and developed an oral method of possibly stripping some of the calcium from the arteries, emulsifying excessive blood fats, cleaning out a little of the lipid deposits, and reducing arterial spasms.

A number of health scientists added to the body of knowledge about oral chelation therapy. Their investigations carried into the realm of perfecting formulations that behave as adjunctives to intravenous injections with ethylene diamine tetraacetic acid in replacing valuable lost minerals for the patient receiving IV treatment. Sometimes these formulations are taken by the patient even before he begins his series of chelation therapy injections. They build his cardiovascular system and tone blood vessel walls in preparation for accepting greater volumes of IV fluids.

Other oral chelate formulations help the chelated patient remain on a maintenance program of high dosage vitamins, minerals, amino acids, enzymes, mucopolysaccharides, herbs, protomorphogens, fiber, hormones, antioxidants, fatty acids, concentrated food molecules, some pharmaceuticals, and other ingredients.

Finally, the researchers have advanced into the area of preventive oral chelates. We are just entering this stage. Oral chelating agents are being introduced to the masses of people now as a medical prevention technique against an individual's gradual but ongoing series of pathological changes in his arteries known as "atherosclerosis" or the ripening state of his cells that we call "aging" or the mutagenic alterations of his cellular genetic material designated as "cancer." Preventive oral chelation therapy is valuable for holding off most degenerative diseases.

If a patient is symptomatically ill with a cardiovascular disorder or other degenerative disease, however, it must be emphasized, and it is so emphatically articulated by every health professional knowledgeable about chelation therapy whom I have queried, that *oral chelation therapy is no substitute for intravenous chelation therapy*. Such an affirmation is particularly true when fast healing time is a factor. For a person in cardiovascular crisis, for example, it's not likely that he or she has the months or years left to wait for oral chelation therapy to reverse accumulated damage to the vascular system. A life or limb in danger requires IV chelation therapy. Perhaps oral chelation therapy will be instituted after the body part is restored and after maintenance care is in order.

More often than not, experiences among chelating physicians indicate that oral chelates take at least eight times longer to show patient health benefits than do IV chelates. Those doctors who have been forced to replace IV chelation therapy in their practices with oral chelation therapy because of medical-legal-political pressure from opponents, such as those in Arizona and Kansas, report that there is no surrogate for the infusion method of administration.

Much greater quantities of chelate for faster and greater benefits can be taken by the patient during an IV sitting. In the spring of 1983, I received 100 grams of vitamin C intravenously in two and a half hours. As a weak organic acid, vitamin C is an excellent chelator. If, instead, I had swallowed 100 grams of vitamin C during that short period, the amount of gastrointestinal upset, including diarrhea, gut spasm, internal gas, and vomiting that would have struck, most likely would have dehydrolyzed me and racked me unto death.

Between variable intervals of booster injections for preventive IV chelation therapy, I regularly ingest oral chelating agents. What am

I attempting to accomplish by my use of various types of product brands of oral chelates? Chelation therapy is a vital function that is taking place in my body already. It does so in all living organisms—plants, animals, bacteria, viruses, yeasts, molds, etc. In your body and mine, chelation forms and then catalyzes into functioning enzymes, amino acids, hormones, and other necessary substances for sustaining life and maintaining health. I am merely helping the process along. I try to find or create those conditions that can benefit my body.

So many environmental disadvantages that we can do nothing about strike all of us every day. Taking oral chelating agents, for me, becomes one small leverage against the pathogens, carcinogens, mutagens, atherogens, allergens, and other body destroyers we must face. Besides avoiding such body abuses as smoking, imbibing alcohol, lacking exercise, obesity, drug-taking, eating additives, drinking impure water, ingesting heavy metals, consuming caffeine, devouring fat, breathing bad air, exhausting endocrines, dissipating strength, and misspending youth, is there any other way to get an edge on surroundings that would pull you down? Popping down my daily quota of oral chelates is a technique that allows me to fight for my life and health more effectively.

It's anticipated that orally administered chelating agents are reducing the elevated incidence of abnormal platelet formation, a condition especially common in patients showing signs of heart disease. The agents also dilate the arteries, enhance cellular ability to utilize oxygen, hold off clotting too quickly by fibrinogen, discourage clumping by red blood cells, reduce elevated serum cholesterol, elasticize arterial walls, allow for the passage of greater blood volume through the vessels, and provide multitudinous means for life extension.

CELLULAR HOMEOSTASIS FROM ORAL CHELATION THERAPY

The idea of a person being whole and at the peak of his chronological powers has recently been popularized by the term "holistic health." Existing in a state of holism is well-being at the macro-level where it's able to be seen by others and felt by yourself. But there is another form of holism that never gets discussed or even acknowl-

edged by people, mainly because it functions at the micro-level—
the level of the cell. Bioinorganic scientists such as Bruce Halstead,
M.D., have described such a microscopic holistic state as "cellular
homeostasis." Homeostasis is equilibrium or a balance between op-
posing pressures in the cell with respect to various functions and to
the chemical composition of its fluids. When practically all cells in a
tissue, organ, or system are homeostatic, that body part is considered to be in optimal health.

"It's a sad fact of natural law," writes Dr. Halstead in *The Scientific
Basis of EDTA Chelation Therapy*, "that all systems have a tendency
toward increasing disorder. The more orderly the arrangement of
matter, in this instance cellular homeostasis, the less likely it is to be
maintained if energy is not expended to counteract the tendency
toward disorder. . . . Living cells are improbable and are inherently
unstable organizations. Maintenance of cellular organization is de-
pendent upon energy that is absorbed from the environment and
transformed into chemical energy. This chemical energy is used to
meet the requirements for the biosynthesis of cellular components,
the osmotic work required to transport materials in and out of the
cell, and myriads of other cellular functions."

Energy-related molecular interactions bring about a continual
chain of events among interdependent cellular reactions when one's
autonomic nervous system or voluntary nervous system meets
some obstacle to its homeostasis, such as inhaling exhaust fumes
from a diesel-powered bus. Enzyme catalysts come into play.
Chemical-bond energy from your body's adenosine triphosphate
(ATP), the universal energy currency of all living organisms, causes
a series of reactant cells to "rev their engines" and counter the
obstacle-stimulus with appropriate enzyme secretions. This engine-
revving probably takes place among your cells a million times during each waking period, and to a lesser extent during sleep. That's
why you can get away with meeting 10,000 pollutants while walking through a major city's traffic-snarled streets. Indeed, enzymes
that are needed by your body to counteract newly introduced pollutants are invented by your cells in mini-seconds. Oral chelating
agents are required for continuing such spontaneous invention.

Dr. Halstead says, "In atherosclerosis there is a progressive di-
minishment of some of the vital arterial enzyme systems due to
calcium deposition, and the build-up of biochemical lesions and

non-soluble substrates. It is the impairment of this energy currency exchange which plays a vital role in the pathogenesis of atherosclerosis. Thus, atherosclerosis is essentially a clinical reflection of the Second Law of Thermodynamics."

Thermodynamics is the branch of physics dealing with energy and its transformations. The Second Law of Thermodynamics states that physical and chemical processes always proceed with an increase in the disorder of randomness. Physicists call such random disorder "entropy."

Previously I quoted Dr. Halstead as saying that homeostasis will break down unless the cell continuously expends energy to counter the tendency toward disorder. Where will the cell get its energy? From the food you eat. Yet it's well known among holistic nutritionists that much of the food consumed in industrialized Western countries is devitalized from overprocessing and from truck farming's overchemicalization. How can you supplement your diet with nutrients that are missing from devitalized foods? Taking oral chelating agents on a regular basis is a marvelous way to subtly thumb one's nose at the food processor and big industrial agriculturist who would exploit the supermarket shopper by selling malnourishment.

OFFSETTING FREE RADICAL PATHOLOGY

Johan Bjorksten, Ph.D., research director of the Bjorksten Research Foundation in Madison, Wisconsin, is in favor of one's consumption of oral chelating agents. Dr. Bjorksten is the developer of the crosslinkage theory of aging. The crosslinkage theory holds that aging is caused by single atoms of protein crosslinking with nucleic acid molecules. One of the ways this happens is that free radicals within the organism uncouple from their attachments, get exceedingly excited, become highly reactive, and smash their way into other atoms.

Free radicals have odd numbers of electrons; their orbits are unfilled with paired electrons. Ordinarily, atoms with filled orbits are stable and have paired electrons spinning in opposite directions to balance each other's magnetic movements. An unbalanced situation results when a pair of electrons are separated by your drawing in cigarette smoke, submitting yourself to an X-ray examination, basking in the sun, eating a bologna sandwich, drinking a cocktail, and taking on other forms of self-abuse. The result of free radical impacts in your body will be lipid peroxidation damage to intracellular membranes, outright destruction of cells and maybe whole groups of cells, the formation of chronic degenerative diseases such as liver dysfunction or blindness, and a giant step in the direction of crosslinkage with less time left on your biological clock. The main pathological process that terminates from all of these deleterious changes is hardening of the arteries.

Each cell is comprised of organelles that are bound inside by membranes, and each organelle performs a metabolic function for the cell such as digestion, waste removal, transporting fluids, delivering power, and other items. When free radicals slam into the organelles' intracellular membranes, they create a destruction and loss of organization of cellular enzymes. There is a disturbance in the nutrient distribution system for the cell and cellular metabolism goes awry. Eventually the cells dies. When enough cells die, signs and symptoms of degenerative disease become obvious. The entire destructive process that I have just described is know as "lipid peroxidation."

The numerous types of oral and intravenous chelating agents aid in inhibiting lipid peroxidation by removing metallic ions required for the process to proceed. In other words, over time, nutrient ingredients taken as food supplements tend to bind on to the metallic ions in ways similar to EDTA. They don't perform their inhibiting actions as quickly as EDTA—in perhaps three years instead of four months—but they do eventually achieve inhibition of lipid peroxidation. And, unless the patient continues to expose himself to body-abusive conditions, the cessation and reversal of lipid peroxidation is maintained. Some of the oral chelating agents that maintain intracellular membrane integrity are selenium, vitamin E, vitamin C, cysteine, methionine, glutathione peroxidase, and many others, which I will discuss beginning in the next chapter.

Writing in the June 1980 issue of *Rejuvenation*, Volume 8, Number 2, the Official Journal of the International Association on the Artificial Prolongation of the Human Specific Lifespan, Donald G. Carpenter, Ph.D., of Calhan, Colorado, in his article, "Correction of Biological Aging," says: "In approximately 90 percent of the cases, death due to arteriosclerosis-produced vascular insufficiency is now avoidable. Furthermore, clinical evidence reveals that the arteriosclerotic deposits can be, and are being, removed by appropriate treatment." Among the treatments that Dr. Carpenter recommends are various forms of chelation therapy.

THE NEED TO REPLACE TOXIC MINERALS
WITH NUTRIENT MINERALS

Dr. Bjorksten in his article "Possibilities and Limitations of Chelation as a Means of Life Extension," published in the September 1980 issue of *Rejuvenation*, Volume 8, Number 3, warns, "The need for aluminum removal is rapidly moving toward the center of gerontological attention . . . [because] of aluminum accumulation paralleling severe mental disturbances in patients in chronic treatment on artificial kidney the immunohisto-chemical relationship between Alzheimer fibrillary tangles and aluminum-induced filaments and the detection of focal accumulations of aluminum and silicon within neurofibrillary tangle-bearing neurons of Alzheimer's disease. Such widely differing diseases as Parkinson's disease and Down's syndrome have also been associated with elevated aluminum content [in the brain]."

In simpler form, Dr. Bjorksten indicates that aluminum toxicity is a potential root cause of Alzheimer's disease, Parkinson's disease, and Down's syndrome, and later in his article he worries about heavy metals bringing on other degenerative diseases.

Research conducted over the last six years by William J. Walsh and fellow analytical chemists at the Argonne National Laboratories has revealed that extremely violent people have abnormal patterns of trace metals in their hair that can be used like chemical fingerprints to identify those who are violence-prone. "This has tremendous possibilities for crime prevention," said Walsh. "It appears that you may be able to predict if a person is prone toward violence by a chemical analysis of his hair."

A simple matter of correcting the violent person's body chemistry would tend to empty our prisons and restore to society people whose neurons malfunctioned because of twisted mineral metabolism. Oral chelating agents could be the replacement for jailhouses. A criminal with the startling violence-prone syndrome like the 13-year-old boy from the little town of McHenry, Illinois, who had been plagued by outbursts of violence, attempting to murder two youths and failing in school as well, no doubt would require intra-venous chelation therapy at first, later to be replaced with oral chelating agents for acceptable societal maintenance.

Argonne National Laboratories scientists began studying trace metals in hair to determine what they could reveal about people's health and behavior. They analyzed more than 60,000 hair samples. One of the first groups to be compared with the normal baseline that the chemists established was composed of ninety-six extremely violent people. Half were inmates at Stateville and Menard prisons in Illinois, and the other half were former convicts and violent children. They represented all races and socioeconomic levels. All the subjects had deliberately and repeatedly hurt other human beings.

Of these violence-prone individuals, 97 percent could be divided into one of two groups based on specific patterns of trace metals in their hair samples, said analytical chemist Walsh. The key trace metals were copper, sodium, and zinc. The "psychotic criminals," who are normal much of the time but suffer episodes of violence, had higher levels of copper, lower levels of zinc, and low levels of sodium in their hair samples.

The "sociopaths," career criminals who are constantly prone to violence, had lower levels of copper, higher levels of sodium, and medium levels of zinc. This group included 58 percent of the violent children and 82 percent of the violent adults. These two distinctive trace metal patterns were identical in blacks, Hispanics, and whites, and in subjects from inner cities, wealthy suburbs, and rural areas, said Walsh. The psychotics and sociopaths also had high levels of lead and cadmium and low levels of cobalt and lithium.

"This is giving us a key to the root cause of violent crime. It might be more related to chemical imbalances than to psychological or sociological factors. The results strongly suggest that violent crimi-nals have chemical imbalances which adversely impact their behav-ior," the scientist added.

A small number of the violent subjects were treated by Carl C. Pfeiffer, Ph.D., M.D., director of the Brain Bio Center in Princeton, New Jersey. Different forms of oral chelating agents were utilized. "They are all doing beautifully," Dr. Pfeiffer said. "There are major personality changes. The sociopaths, for instance, become nice peo-ple instead of being ferocious all the time."

A report on the Argonne National Laboratory findings was prepared for *Science*, the journal of the American Association for the Advancement of Science. It was co-authored by Ronald Isaacson, a former research chemist at Argonne Laboratories who is now with the Gas Research Institute.

THE CLASSIC CASE OF GANGRENE REVERSAL

In the annals of medicine, numbers of patient case histories stand out, and for chelation therapy it is no different. The classic case of diabetic gangrene reversal, used by me in two other books, deserves repeating. It's the case that startles anyone because of the photographs accompanying the patient's record. Photographs were used in *Chelation Therapy* (Freelance Communications, 484 High Ridge Road, Stamford, CT 06905, 1984), but not in *The Chelation Answer* (M. Evans & Co., 216 East 49th Street, New York, NY 10017, 1982). It's the case that set a precedent for the treatment of diabetic gangrene. Heretofore the process of gangrene was not reversible. But now, with administration of chelation therapy, it is.

The treatment has saved the limbs of over 950 patients who were scheduled to have their lower limbs cut off but did not require amputation because they received chelation therapy instead.

The following description is the classic case of gangrene reversal:

After enjoying an outing in very hot weather during the fall of 1975, Roland C. Hohnbaum, D.C., now deceased, who was then 54 years old, practicing as a chiropractic doctor in Richmond, California, noticed that an ulcer had developed on his left foot. Such an ulcer was highly dangerous for Dr. Hohnbaum, since he was a long-term diabetic. Even with knowledge of the ramifications of diabetic ulcers, the chiropractor told himself, "This can't happen to me. I'm different!" But he was not different, and the gangrenous course of arteriosclerosis complicated by diabetes began its insidious creep from his toes upward.

"It developed worse and worse, and finally I was forced down and was flat on my back for about two months," said Dr. Hohnbaum. "I had an internist at the Alta Bates Hospital in Berkeley, California, in whom I had a lot of confidence. He took care of my case in the beginning, but then he became frightened too, saying that I'd have to go to the hospital because I was going to lose my toes."

Also quite frightened himself, Dr. Hohnbaum made a concentrated effort and took hold of his thinking. He decided against amputation for gangrene, since he knew that a decision to operate just *started* at the toes. Gangrene is known to slowly and steadily spread and eventually may require amputation below the knee, above the knee, or even at mid-thigh. Besides, the combination of hardening of the arteries and diabetes were by now showing effects in his other foot too. It meant possibly having both feet cut off.

Because he refused hospitalization and surgery, Dr. Hohnbaum was denied further treatment by both his internist and the consulting vascular surgeon. Afflicted as he was, the patient had to engage in his own self-help program at home by bringing in dietary factors and anything else he could use to improve his health. He prayed that his condition might begin to show some improvement.

"I finally found out about Dr. Tang with the chelation therapy," the chiropractor said while tears formed in his eyes, "and this was a lifesaver for me. I don't think that I can say any more than that I—I have feet under me now."

When Dr. Hohnbaum visited Yiwen Y. Tang, M.D., F.A.B.F.P., of San Francisco, he arrived on crutches and in pain. "The patient was in immediate need of amputation of his two legs below the knee. (See Figure 9.1.) His life was in imminent danger. He could bear nothing on his feet—not hosiery—certainly not shoes," Dr. Tang told me. Dr. Tang supplied me with the photographs that depict the condition of Dr. Hohnbaum's feet on these pages. After careful diagnostic studies, Dr. Tang began Dr. Hohnbaum on chelation treatments.

"The pre-chelation tests also indicated clogging of my carotid artery, making me a prime target for stroke," said Dr. Roland Hohnbaum.

Within a week of having the first treatment, the patient could put on socks. (See Figure 9.1.) By January 1976, two months after the last of fifteen chelations, he wore shoes and returned to work full time. The chiropractor is now completely healed with no evidence of anything having happened to his feet.

"Post-chelation tests show my carotid arteries now clear of occlusion. There is no doubt that the atherosclerosis which had accompanied my diabetes had been abated," Dr. Hohnbaum concluded.

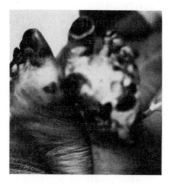

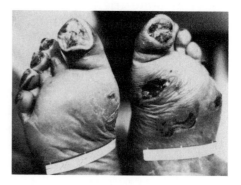

1. Just two days prior to Dr. Hohn-baum's scheduled operation for amputation because of the presence of diabetic gangrene and ulcerations (October 23, 1975). He could bear nothing on his feet—not even hosiery—because of the pain. The dead black areas on his feet indicate that under usual medical procedure, he had been properly directed to have both limbs cut off just below the knees.

2. Just one week following the first treatment with chelation therapy administered by Dr. Tang to the patient, Dr. Hohnbaum, the ulcerated areas are beginning to heal in from the edges and the gangrene has reversed itself. Here, October 30, 1975, the diabetic is able to wear hosiery. His pain is gone.

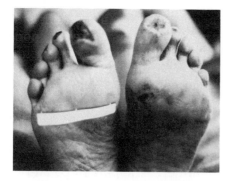

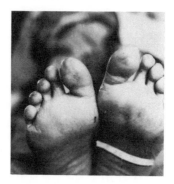

3. Two months after the last of fifteen chelation treatments, in January 1976, Dr. Hohnbaum wore shoes and returned to work full time. His diabetic gangrene was eliminated completely and the ulcerations were almost completely healed.

4. Shown are the chiropractor's feet March 28, 1976, when there no longer are signs of the gangrene and ulcerations. Chelation therapy has reversed the gangrenous process and reduced hardening of the arteries to his lower extremities. The patient has avoided bilateral leg amputation.

Figure 9.1.   Improvement in Dr. Hohnbaum's feet due to chelation therapy.

Dr. Hohnbaum's case and more than 950 others like his have changed medical thinking in this country about diabetic gangrene. Previously thought to have been irreversible, diabetic ulcers and gangrene now can be cured by chelation therapy.

Roland Hohnbaum added a postscript to his story. He said, "I am still haunted by the flat statement made to me by a vascular surgeon whom I had met after my feet were all healed. Upon seeing the photographs of my gangrenous feet, the surgeon told me, 'If you had been my patient and your feet looked like these pictures, there is no question—I would have amputated.'"

A couple of years later, my wife and I met Dr. and Mrs. Hohnbaum quite by coincidence in Dr. Tang's San Francisco office (just before the physician moved to Reno, Nevada, to escape the terrible harassment he had been experiencing from organized medicine). As it happens, Hohnbaum visited Dr. Tang once a year for a series of booster injections with EDTA and to have his oral chelating agents reevaluated to make sure he was taking the appropriate nutritional supplements and other food chelators that make up a part of his lifestyle. Because I had utilized the patient's case history and his photographs of gangrenous feet in my books, out of appreciation I invited the couple to join my wife and me at dinner. They declined because of a prior commitment, part of their regular weekly schedule. Mrs. Hohnbaum told us that the two of them were on their way to an evening of ballroom dancing. "You see, Dr. Walker," the woman said with a smile, "Roland loves to dance."

CHAPTER TEN
The Chelation Diet and Its Foods

According to exercise physiologists and medical researchers who have examined him, Noel Johnson of San Diego, California, is a modern-day "superman." At age 90, Mr. Johnson has slowed his aging process to such an extent that doctors say he is in better physical condition than many men forty years his junior.

"He's running against Father Time, and winning," one admiring physician says.

Indeed, Johnson competes in foot races and boxing matches worldwide, and has a standing challenge to outrun or outpunch anyone over sixty-five years old. "I'm the only man in the world who does what I do. No one can compete with me," says Johnson, who pulls no punches in his statements, but may not be entirely correct. "Some people talk and write extensively about health and fitness, but I'll outlive them all."

The President's Council on Physical Fitness and Sports was so impressed by the man's prowess that it made Johnson the guest of honor at the Presidential Sports/Fitness Festival held in Minneapolis, September 10, 1983. The Council believed that Johnson's active lifestyle, his nutrition program, and his youthful attitude are just the examples that millions of Americans need to shed excess pounds and huff and puff their way back to health.

Indeed, this senior sportsperson did steal the show. He was a man who once suffered with heart trouble, arthritis, bursitis, gout, and impotence. Now he has become one of America's medical marvels.

There are no secrets, says Johnson, who wrote a book in 1982 entitled, appropriately enough, *A Dud at 70, a Stud at 80!* The fellow reasons that if he, at age 70, could start life anew, so can anyone else.

Until 1969, Johnson led a sedentary existence. "My wife was a vegetable with psychotic senility, lying in the hospital after several strokes. I was just retired and spending the time at home doing nothing. Smoking. Drinking beer. My doctor told me I shouldn't even push a lawnmower or I might die. I was a wreck and about forty pounds overweight," he recalls.

Feeling ambitious one afternoon, Johnson went out on a quarter-mile track with his son for some overdue exercise and found that he couldn't run a hundred feet. So poor was his condition, in fact, that his son wanted to put him in a convalescent home where he could receive proper care during his last days on earth. "That suggestion made me a little peeved," the elderly man says.

A prizefighter in his younger days, Johnson decided it was time to get in shape. And that he did. Exercise became a daily routine, and though at first he could not complete even one lap around the track without gasping for air, he ran a marathon two years after beginning training.

The exercise that Noel Johnson does is chelating his body naturally. Johan Bjorksten, Ph.D., a world famous authority on life extension, recommends that one use his muscles for lactic acid production, for lactic acid is the body's own chelating agent. "It is an established fact that the lactic acid or lactate content of the blood is about doubled during the time of moderate muscular exertion," writes Dr. Bjorksten in *Rejuvenation*. "Since lactic acid is a good chelating agent, it may help remove from the system potentially crosslinking aluminum, cadmium, mercury, lead, arsenic, and excess iron, among others, thereby increasing longevity if depletion of the needed chelatable metals manganese, cobalt, zinc, iron and perhaps molybdenum is counteracted by supplemental medication or a couple quarts daily of skim milk."

Johnson's diet changed also. He began to eat foods that are natural chelation agents such as fresh fruit, fresh vegetables, nuts, seeds, and honeybee pollen (to be discussed in Chapter Twelve). They became substitutes for steaks and hamburgers.

"It's remarkable what he's done for himself," says Dr. Jack Wilmore, a University of Arizona physical education professor and nationally recognized fitness expert, when discussing Noel Johnson. "He's a phenomenal specimen for his age."

Johnson runs between eight and ten marathons annually. He holds several distance running records for men over seventy years old, and is the World Senior Boxing Champion, a title he defended successfully at the Senior Olympics in July 1983. He has also been a champion of a different sort, having appeared on the cover of five million Wheaties packages in 1977.

"When I started this," he says, referring to his new lifestyle, "I thought I would probably peak at 75 or so. But I feel better now than I did at 75, and I expect to keep getting better." So good does he feel that his goal is to live beyond 100.

"I see no reason why I can't live to be even 150," Johnson says. "We can create our own destiny. We determine what happens, choose health or illness. It's what I call creative thinking. Not just thinking 'I should do this,' but thinking it and then creating it in your life. Make it happen."

Lenore Zohman, M.D., one of the nation's most respected cardiologists, says Johnson "looks like he's in his early sixties, with legs like a man in his thirties." Dr. Zohman put the patient through a series of tests recently at Montefiore Hospital in New York City. "Noel is refuting the misconception that we must decline with age, that aging is degeneration. Diseases in older adults don't have to be accepted as part of the aging process. Heart disease is not necessarily concomitant to getting old," said Dr. Zohman.

Subjecting his 5-foot, 7.5-inch, 135-pound body to the most sophisticated health-measuring tests man can devise, Johnson has set a string of age-group running records, including a 6:27 minute indoor mile and a 3:01 half mile. He is the oldest runner to complete the New York City Marathon. One of his goals is to be the first 100-year-old man to complete a marathon (26.2 miles). (The oldest person on record to complete a marathon is Mr. C. Iordanidis, age 98, who, in 1976, clocked seven hours, thirty-three minutes.)

Johnson gets some of his exercise these days on the dance floor, preferring ballroom and square dancing to the disco variety. It has helped bring him an active and interesting social life. When he was asked a few days before I wrote this the last time he had sex with a woman, Johnson looked at his watch and replied: "About three hours ago." If he is partial to younger women (he is widowed), it is only because few gals his age can keep up with him. "I don't care if they're eighteen or eighty," he mentioned, "so long as they can run, dance, or are good in bed."

What is the secret of Noel Johnson's amazing youthfulness, even though he's ninety years old? He chelates himself at home every day as a preventive measure against developing any degenerative disease. His self-chelation technique comes naturally out of the exercise program and chelation diet that he follows. His current exercise program involves an easy run for ninety minutes, five days each week. In addition to taking bee pollen tablets, he is especially enthusiastic about eating raw foods, such as live seeds and foliage—green leaves that capture the sun and the energy of the universe. He is fond of lemon leaves and seeds that germinate. "If it doesn't germinate, it's dead, and a person needs live seeds to keep his cells alive," he says. One of Johnson's maxims is: "If you have to cook it, overlook it."

THE CHELATION DIET

M. Paul Dommers, M.D., of Belvidere, Illinois, sets down guidelines for his patients when he wants them to follow the chelation diet. The following is what Dr. Dommers advises:

- Cut your intake of white and brown sugars; you may use honey, measured at the equivalent of ¼ cup of honey to one cup of sugar.
- Use whole grain flours such as whole wheat or rye. If you must use white flour, make sure it is unbleached.
- Eat baked potatoes including the skins; never put French fries into your mouth.
- Use only whole grain cereals and breads in your diet.
- Reduce salt intake to a minimum. If you must use salt, take sea salt or Lite salt in place of regular.
- You may use the equivalent of one to two pats of butter per day, but not margarine. Only lightly utilize corn oil, olive oil, saf-

flower oil, or sesame seed oil.
- Avoid hydrogenated fats of any type including shortening such as Crisco. Don't eat peanut butter that is hydrogenated. Avoid eating store-bought cakes or pies, cookies, rolls, biscuits, crackers, doughnuts, pizza, and pretzels. Unless they are made from whole wheat or spinach or artichoke, eliminate pasta. Absolutely do away with white flour macaroni, spaghetti, and noodles from your diet.
- Minimize your use of caffeine products such as regular tea, coffee, chocolate, and the various cola beverages. You may drink decaffeinated beverages, Sanka, and most herb teas.
- Avoid store-bought milks and milk products if raw milk is available. (Dr. Dommers practices in the milk-capital region of the United States.) Eat yogurt, but not the fruit-flavored type. Do not use processed cheeses; use natural cheeses only, especially those classified as "aged" cheeses.
- You may have from four to six eggs per week, but they should be soft- or hard-boiled or poached. Don't scramble eggs unless you do it in a microwave oven.
- Never eat processed luncheon-type meats such as sausage, frankfurters, and any other products that contain nitrites. Avoid salami and bologna at all costs.
- Get your animal protein from fish and poultry and not from pork, beef, and mutton. Chicken and turkey are particularly recommended but be sure to remove the skin from all poultry. Roast, boil, or bake poultry and fish; never fry these foods.
- Nut meats are also a good source of protein. Almonds, walnuts, and other nuts (but not macadamia nuts or peanuts) are allowed. Pumpkin seeds, sunflower seeds, and other seed types are acceptable. Never eat salted nuts or salted seeds. Use the more natural nut butters with no dextrose sugar or hydrogenation added. These natural nut butters must be refrigerated after you have opened them.
- Increase your fluid intake with good, pure spring water, filtered water, or other water that does not come directly from the tap. Drink a minimum of six to eight glasses of water each day. You can also take fluids in the form of vegetable and fruit juices, but these must be of the unsweetened type.
- Fresh green-leafed vegetables, such as spinach, and fresh or

ange-colored vegetables, such as carrots, are excellent complex carbohydrate types of foods. Obtain romaine lettuce when possible and eat a wide variety of vegetables. Steam them or eat them raw; do not overcook them.

- Eat some fruit each day; between meals is a good time for snacking on fruits.
- Take your daily supplements for oral chelation therapy as directed by the doctor.
- Follow an approved daily exercise program and reduce your overweight.

There is not one menu plan for the chelation diet. A number of investigators have put forth eating programs that could be adapted for their anti-atherosclerotic effect. Michio Kushi's standard macrobiotic diet might be modified for the purposes of a chelation lifestyle. Nathan Pritikin, now deceased, advocated an excellent menu plan with appropriate recipes. The hypoglycemic diet could be used for chelation purposes. The items that are missing in all of these healthful menu plans, however, are particular foods and food supplements that are known oral chelators. I will begin discussing them in the next section.

For now, a generally recommended eating program to follow consists of the following chelation diet:

- Whole cereal grains should comprise about 25 percent of overall food consumption. Whole grains include brown rice, millet, whole wheat, oats, rye, corn, barley, and buckwheat. Preferably you should eat such grains as the meal's main course or as a side dish. They may be mixed and matched for flavor and consistency. You can also take them in the form of floured products such as rice cakes, whole wheat bread, rye bread, corn bread, or another good-tasting, dark, non-caramel-colored whole grain bread.
- One or two cups of soup, thick with fresh vegetables, brown rice, and containing some seaweed, may be eaten as a filler at each meal. Soups may be made from beans, whole grains, miso, tofu, tomato, or have a poultry frame as the basis for its stock.
- Fresh vegetables should comprise approximately 25 percent of the daily food intake. Such steamed, wok'd, sautéed, or raw

vegetables as green cabbage, kale, collard and mustard greens, Swiss chard, watercress, bok choy, dandelion, burdock root, carrots, radishes, turnips, onions, acorn squash, Hubbard squash, butternut squash, cauliflower, zucchini, broccoli, beets, celery, mushrooms, eggplant, potatoes, asparagus, spinach, sweet potatoes, yams, green and red peppers, and others that are locally grown are good eating for stimulating self-chelation therapy.

- About 10 percent of your daily food consumption should include cooked beans and sea vegetables. Typical beans you may prefer are garbanzo, lima, pinto, black, lentils, red, kidney, and the soybean products of *azuki*, *tempeh*, and *natto*. Mineral-rich sea vegetables for soups and side dishes might be dulse, Irish moss, *alaria*, *hijiki*, *kombu*, *wakame*, and *nori*.
- Animal protein could comprise 25 percent of the chelation diet. White meat fish and white meat poultry are preferred over blue skin or red meat varieties of animal flesh.
- Fresh fruit should make up the balance of calories and be nearly 15 percent of the diet's bulk. Never add flavorings to fresh fruit such as salt on watermelon or sugar on grapefruit. These white additives destroy the value of the food. You might try squeezing lime on honeydew or lemon on cantaloupe, however.

The chelation diet is not a reducing diet. It isn't concerned with calories, and no restrictions in quantity exist. The major matter of interest for the chelation diet and what makes it different from any other is its focus on bringing specific nutrients either as whole foods or as food supplements into the overall eating program.

NUTRIENTS THAT ACT AS CHELATORS

In your own kitchen, you can demonstrate the process of chelation therapy carried on by particular foods. Accumulate some eggshells, which are loaded with calcium. (In fact eggshells often are utilized in the industrial process of creating a calcium supplement.) Let the shells lie in a cup of vinegar over a number of days. As time passes, you will notice that the shells are getting thinner and thinner until they finally disappear. What has happened is that the vinegar, which is acetic acid, a weak organic acid that acts as an excellent chelator, has chelated the calcium right out of the eggshell and dissolved it into an ionic form.

When oral chelates carry out this same sort of eggshell process for metastatic calcium deposited in the body, such reconstituted calcium once again becomes useful for employment by the parathyroid gland. The oral chelates take metastatic calcium out of deposits in the arteries, arthritic joints, bursae, and cell structures where it does not belong and put it into the blood stream in charged ionic form. The metastatic calcium apatite no longer poses a danger to your health. Once again ionic calcium becomes beneficial for building teeth and bones, strengthening cell membranes, preventing muscular and arterial spasms, and other good purposes.

Medical researchers have found that those patients suffering from heart disease show degrees of deficiency in the following descending order of three particular nutrients: vitamin E, the mineral selenium, and vitamin C. Additionally, people having some cardiovascular defects lack the proper amounts of magnesium, manganese, zinc, chromium, and potassium. These missing minerals are best supplemented into the diet with salts of ascorbate, aspartate, and/or orotate.

A number of other food supplements function as oral chelating agents as well. Among these different food chelators are any of the edible weak organic acids, such as lactic acid, acetic acid, ascorbic acid, and citric acid; lecithin; fiber; the oxygenator N, N-dimethylglycine; spirulina; bee pollen; particular amino acids such as L-cysteine; the bioflavonoids including rutin; all of the B-complex vitamins; certain other minerals, such as iodine, iron, germanium, and silicon; particular protomorphogens including adrenal substance and thymus; some rather vital herbs like garlic; a few enzymes including bromelain and papain; and numbers of assorted items, such as omega-3 fatty acids. The balance of this chapter and all of the next will provide brief discussions of selected examples of these various food supplements.

Vitamin E (tocopherol) is a fat-soluble vitamin composed of a group of seven compounds called alpha, beta, delta, epsilon, eta, gamma, and zeta tocopherols. They occur in highest concentrations in cold-pressed vegetable oils such as wheat germ, all whole raw seeds and nuts, and soybeans. It is an antioxidant, preventing saturated fatty acids and vitamin A from combining with other harmful substances, and protecting the B-complex vitamins from oxidizing when present in the digestive tract.

What makes vitamin E a chelating agent is its ability to unite with oxygen and stop it from converting into various peroxides so that the red blood cells are left free to carry oxygen to body parts. Thus, cellular respiration of all muscle fibers, especially the cardiac and skeletal fibers, may function with less oxygen. This phenomenon increases the muscle fibers' stamina and endurance. Vitamin E also dilates the blood vessels to increase blood flow, acts against thromboxin to inhibit clot formation, and strengthens capillary membranes to protect them from destruction by poisons such as serum hydrogen peroxide. It promotes linoleic acid production, retards cellular aging, helps the eyes focus, and prevents both the pituitary and adrenal hormones from oxidizing. Vitamin E acts as a diuretic, reduces cardiac edema, holds down high blood pressure after it is brought under control by medication, and protects against environmental toxins such as radiation.

One of the best sources of vitamin E is offered by the A. C. Grace Company of Big Sandy, Texas. Company President R. Erickson furnishes all-natural unesterified vitamin E in 400 IU bovine soft gel capsules that provide full antioxidant, antithrombic, anti-fatigue, and anti-scar effectiveness. This vitamin E has high antidote quality against free radical pathology. There is no artificial color, preservatives, or flavor added. You may contact the A. C. Grace Company at Route 2, Box 193, Carrington Lane, Big Sandy, Texas 75755; telephone (214) 636-4368.

Wilfrid Shute, M.D., and Evan Shute, M.D., at the Shute Institute for Clinical and Laboratory Medicine in London, Ontario, Canada, have recommended the daily use of 800 to 1600 international units (IU) of vitamin E. Richard Passwater, Ph.D., reports that he received 20,000 replies to a survey he had conducted through *Prevention* magazine stating that vitamin E gradually improved angina, circulatory problems, leg pains, and irregular heartbeat in the magazine's readers. Dr. Passwater said that 400 IU taken for a minimum of ten years seemed to be the most popular dosage range of vitamin E protection. Most holistic physicians agree with this estimate and say that the vitamin is the best preventive for blood clots, as the natural vitamin E has no specific injurious side effects.

Selenium is a trace mineral antioxidant that works well with vitamin E to enhance its metabolic reactions. It acts as a chelating agent by delaying oxidation of polyunsaturated fatty acids that can cause solidification of tissue proteins. Thus, selenium tends to preserve elasticity of the tissues, especially the arterial walls. It is most often found in the germ and bran of cereals, in vegetables such as broccoli, onions, and tomatoes, and in tuna fish. A usual food supplement dosage is in the vicinity of 100 micrograms (mcg) to 300 micrograms per day.

Vitamin C (ascorbic acid) is a water-soluble vitamin, unstable in the presence of oxygen, light, heat, and air, which stimulates the activity of oxidative enzymes. Since it's a weak organic acid and has antioxidant properties, it is a good oral chelating agent and IV chelating agent. Metabolically, vitamin C catalyzes the actions of the amino acids phenylalanine and tyrosine, converts the inactive form of folic acid to the active folinic acid, protects thiamine, riboflavin, pantothenic acid, and vitamins A and E against oxidation, and stimulates calcium metabolism. It is present in most fresh fruits and vegetables, and its dietary supplements may be prepared from rose hips, acerola cherries, green peppers, and citrus fruits. A usual food supplement dosage varies greatly according to patient tolerance and need, but it seems to range from 1,000 milligrams to 6,000 milligrams per day.

Vitamin C deficiency tends to bring on a loss of particular chemical substances in blood vessels, which results in roughening and irregularity of the walls. Here is where atherosclerotic plaque may begin, thereby forming circulatory clogging. It is necessary to supplement with vitamin C or to eat larger quantities of foods containing ascorbic acid, because a necessary enzyme that is missing in the human liver prevents us from manufacturing our own. One vital duty of white blood cells is to carry vitamin C in the bloodstream. After a heart attack, the victim's heart begins to heal aided by an elevation of ascorbic acid. R. Hume, M.D., of Glasgow, Scotland, discovered that the vitamin is drawn from the blood to renew cardiac fiber repair and to rebuild collagen.

The **ascorbates** are chemical salt derivatives of ascorbic acid which are created when the vitamin reacts in the bloodstream with magnesium to form magnesium ascorbate, zinc to form zinc ascorbate, calcium to form calcium ascorbate, etc. Therefore, one really should not discuss vitamin C without a follow-up description of the ascorbates.

When it is desired by the physician to intravenously chelate his patient with ascorbic acid, it is administered as an ascorbate. This vitamin C salt is used because the doctor knows that the vitamin by itself is not tolerated well by the blood vessels and the body's blood chemistry, in general.

Vitamin C, taken orally as calcium, magnesium, selenium, sodium, potassium, manganese, and/or zinc ascorbates, provides a more absorbable and more soluble product. Vitamin C acts as a chelating agent for the minerals. Dr. Passwater has learned that oral mineral ascorbates taken for their vitamin C content are better tolerated by critically ill people than straight ascorbic acid.

Dr. Robert Downs, in an article written by Alice Van Baak and published in *Bestways*, describes the chelating action of vitamin C when taken by mouth. Dr. Downs says: "Taken at normal dosages, this vitamin will not cause any problem chelating or wasting minerals because the absorption and transport systems of the body can handle several grams a day with no trouble. . . . In taking normal doses of vitamin C, the body systems and the absorption systems are not under stress, so it doesn't matter what type of vitamin C an individual is taking, but when one needs huge doses of this vitamin, it frequently affects other nutrients. In megadoses this vitamin causes a number of critically-needed minerals to be excreted through the urine. Calcium and magnesium are the most severely hit because our chemicalized soil prevents us from having an adequate amount of these elements in the first place. The diuretic action of vitamin C is the cause of the mineral excretions. If mineral supplements aren't given to replace the stolen minerals, deficiency symptoms appear.

"Doctors and scientists know that vitamin C increases iron absorption," Dr. Downs continued. "It was recently found that it also increases calcium absorption. Obviously, ascorbate absorption is also increased because more ascorbate can be taken before it is rejected by vomiting or diarrhea. Some people absorb only a small part of ascorbate from each dose of ascorbic acid. These people will profit enormously from chelated 'C' if they take the mineral ascorbates instead of continuing with ascorbic acid."

The particular formula for accomplishing oral chelation therapy currently being used in the Dr. Downs technique is composed of the following: ascorbic acid, sodium ascorbate, magnesium ascorbate, zinc ascorbate, manganese ascorbate, selenium ascorbate, potassium aspartate, magnesium aspartate, and potassium citrate. Potassium citrate has a slight blood-thinning action; magnesium ascorbate has an antagonistic effect on calcium deposits; selenium ascorbate puts oxygen into the tissues; zinc and manganese ascorbates are enhancers of fat metabolism; potassium and magnesium aspartates regulate cardiovascular conductivity and assist in removing unwanted metastatic calcium in circulatory pathways. The patient starts taking the formula with one cubic centimeter (cc) dosage daily. The amount is increased over time in 1 cc increments until symptoms of intolerance are experienced, and then the dosage is cut back to the tolerance level where there is no longer diarrhea or nausea. The dosage is kept up for three to six months until the benefits of oral chelation therapy are well established.

Aspartic acid (L-aspartate) goes into the inner layer of the outer membranes of tissue cells to release the magnesium portion of the magnesium aspartate molecule. The magnesium helps to displace the calcium ion that is perpetually attempting to permeate cell walls. L-aspartate is a true chelating substance, derived from the essential amino acid—aspartic acid. Not only does it come combined with magnesium, but it is made into a product also containing potassium aspartate. One source of this material in the United States is Advanced Dietary Products Inc., Carl Staley, President, 119 River Drive, P. O. Box 27883, Tempe, Arizona 85282. Telephone toll free at (800) 528-3333; in Arizona (602) 968-0600.

Using magnesium aspartate and potassium aspartate together, you may experience an increase in your heart pump blood volume and an increase in total energy output. These are important food supplements for athletes desiring to maximize performance during their competitions, as well as for patients with heart disease, including complications from atherosclerosis or vascular spasm. The approximate dosage is 90 milligrams daily of potassium aspartate and 32 milligrams daily of magnesium aspartate.

Holistic physicians utilize the aspartic acid supplemental items, and the information presented here comes from their practical applications. Nothing written in these pages should be accepted as a substitute for your own doctor's advice. What you read written by me in connection with oral chelation therapy, either in *The Chelation Way* or elsewhere, is merely of nutritional interest and is not offered as medical advice.

Orotic acid and the **orotate salts** of calcium, magnesium, and zinc are extremely effective and nontoxic mineral complexes. The therapeutic effect of orotic acid includes decreasing the incidence of necrosis in myocardial infarction, increasing the rate of regeneration of healthy cellular and fibrous connective tissue in the infarct region, and increasing the cardiac mass and work capacity. These effects are attributed to the increased myocardial nucleic acid content and protein synthesis. Calcium orotate, magnesium orotate, and zinc orotate are excellent oral chelating agents. They have been used in the management of neonatal jaundice by reducing bilirubin levels in newborns. A study of eighty adults with myocardial infarction treated with orotic acid allowed no deaths due to heart failure. It has produced partial remission of pernicious anemia. A recent investigation of the orotates for decreasing hyperlipidemia proved successful. The dosage range varies for each mineral orotate: calcium orotate is 300 to 600 milligrams/day; potassium orotate is about 500 to 700 milligrams daily; magnesium orotate ranges at 200 to 600 milligrams/day; zinc orotate is approximately 100 milligrams daily. At this writing, the Food and Drug Administration has objected to claims made for the orotates and has frightened the raw material manufacturers from supplying the products for consumer distribution. However, a ready supply of orotates alone and orotates in combination with aspartates is provided by Advanced Dietary Products Inc., 119 Rivers Drive, P. O. Box 27883, Tempe, Arizona 85282; telephone (602) 968-0600 or (800) 528-3333.

Magnesium dietary deficiency may be the cause of sudden death in patients with ischemic heart disease, according to researchers at Downstate Medical Center in New York. Drs. Burton M. Altura and Prasad D.M.V. Turlapaty believe the lack of magnesium in the diet of people in the Western world may explain the high incidence of heart attack that kills over 600,000 Americans each year. Many of the victims have no evidence of atherosclerosis, coronary thrombosis, or other pathological condition at postmortem. Spasm of the coronary arteries from lower than normal levels of magnesium in the cardiac muscle and coronary vessels is thought to be the cause.

Besides selenium, magnesium is among the most important oral chelating minerals available. It promotes absorption and metabolism of other minerals, such as calcium, phosphorus, sodium, and potassium. It also catalyzes the utilization of the B-complex, C, and E vitamins. Magnesium is necessary for the proper function of the cardiac muscles. Widely distributed in foods, it is found in fresh green vegetables, raw wheat germ, soybeans, figs, corn, apples, seeds, and nuts, especially almonds. When supplementing with magnesium, the usual dosage is 500 milligrams daily.

Manganese is another excellent orally chelating trace mineral at a daily intake of 30 milligrams. It aids in the utilization of choline, thiamine, biotin, and ascorbic acid. It catalyzes the synthesis of fatty acids and necessary cholesterol in the body and helps in producing protein, carbohydrates, and fat for various structures, especially for the skeletal system. It is found in such foods as whole-grain cereals, egg yolks, and green vegetables. Manganese is poorly absorbed in the intestinal tract so that supplementing will not get much of it to stay in the body.

Zinc is the constituent of at least twenty-five enzymes involved in digestion and metabolism, including the enzyme carbonic anhydrase, necessary for tissue respiration. It is the mineral component of insulin, essential in the synthesis of nucleic acid and the normal functioning of the prostate and reproductive organs. It improves wound healing and is required in the synthesis of DNA. The best source of zinc for its oral chelating effect are foods such as brewer's yeast, wheat bran, wheat germ, pumpkin seeds, and sunflower seeds. The usual supplemental daily dose of zinc is 22.5 milligrams.

Vanadium reduces the formation of cholesterol in the human central nervous system when the mineral is taken by mouth. It's usually found in fish and may be supplemented daily with 20 milligrams in the form of vanadium oxide.

Chromium is an enzyme stimulator when the body is involved in the metabolism of glucose for energy and the synthesis of fatty acids and cholesterol. It increases the effectiveness of insulin, transports protein for its binding action with RNA, and is mandatory in the effective functioning of the heart muscle. Food sources include clams, corn oil, whole grains, fruits, vegetables, brewer's yeast, and some meats. The usual daily supplemental dosage for chromium as a good oral chelating agent is 200 micrograms.

Potassium is found in the intracellular and extracellular fluids of the cells, acting as a regulator of water balance. It is necessary for growth, stimulates nerve impulses to contract muscles, and preserves alkalinity of the body fluids. It functions in enzyme reactions, cell metabolism, stimulation of the kidneys, and synthesis of muscle protein. Potassium works with sodium to normalize the heartbeat and nourish the muscular system. Food sources consist of vegetables, especially green leafy ones, oranges, whole grains, sunflower seeds, mint leaves, potatoes, and bananas. The standard daily dosage for potassium supplementation as a good oral chelator is 100 milligrams.

Iodine (iodide) regulates energy, promotes growth and development, stimulates the metabolic rate, burns excess fat, converts carotene to vitamin A, synthesizes protein by means of ribosome action, and aids in the functioning of the thyroid gland. In cardiovascular disease, iodine prevents malfunctioning of the normal fat metabolism into cholesterol, which could collect along arterial walls. Its food sources are the sea vegetables Irish moss and kelp, mushrooms, and sea animals. To supplement with iodine, take a daily dosage of 100 micrograms.

Iron combines with protein and copper to make hemoglobin, which in turn transports oxygen in the blood from the lungs to the tissues. It also helps to build muscle tissue, to promote enzymatic action for protein metabolism, to improve respiratory action, and to increase the body's resistance to stress and disease. Iron's best food sources are liver, oysters, heart, lean meat, leafy green vegetables, and tongue. To supplement with iron, the usual daily dose is 20 milligrams.

Silicon, organically bound to silica for making it absorbable by the gut, is a trace element whose need in human nutrition is not well established and whose U.S. recommended daily allowance has not been determined. Nevertheless, chelating physicians have observed that it has a chelation effect when taken by the patient as part of his or her nutritional program. The usual dosage is 50 micrograms per day.

B-complex vitamins act as oral chelating agents, some more than others. *Niacin (vitamin B-3)* in particular reduces serum cholesterol, high blood pressure, and the pain of cramped leg muscles by improving blood flow. It has a dilation effect that goes into the cell and liberates a natural blood-thinning agent. Please note that the vascular dilating effect of niacin is not duplicated by niacinamide so that niacin is the chelator and not niacinamide. But a dosage of 100 milligrams of niacinamide is useful.

To avoid the discomfort of niacin flush, take small amounts, 50 to 100 milligrams, one to four times daily, rather than large dosages all at once. Increase the smaller doses as tolerance builds until you arrive at 500 milligrams of time-released tablets or capsules three times daily, when the optimal chelating effect is achieved.

All of the B-complex vitamins are vital, but pyridoxine (vitamin B-6) 100 milligrams, riboflavin (vitamin B-2) 50 milligrams, thiamine (vitamin B-1) 50 milligrams, and pantothenic acid (vitamin B-5) 300 milligrams have a greater chelating effect. The doses for the other B-complex vitamins follow: cobalamin (vitamin B-12) 100 micrograms, folic acid 400 micrograms, biotin 400 micrograms, choline 250 milligrams, inositol 200 milligrams, PABA (para-amino benzoic acid) 100 milligrams.

Bioflavonoids (vitamin P) are water soluble and composed of brightly colored food substances usually present in fruits and vegetables as companions to vitamin C. The bioflavonoids consist of citrin, hesperidin, rutin, flavones, and flavonols. Rutin has been established as an oral chelator and helps prevent hemorrhages, ruptures, and disruptions of the capillary beds and connective tissues. The body's utilization of vitamin C is increased when bioflavonoids are present. A usual supplemental dosage of bioflavonoids is 100 milligrams.

All of the preceding chelation-type nutrients can be acquired from the following sources by sending for their catalogues:

Willner Chemists Inc.
Irv Willner, President
330 Lexington Avenue
New York, New York 10016
(212) 685-0448

L and H Vitamins Inc.
Lloyd H. Marmon, President
37-10 Crescent Street
Long Island City, New York 11101
(800) 221-1152 or (718) 937-7400

Freeda and Vitamins Inc.
Philip Zimmerman, Chief Chemist
36 East 41st Street
New York, New York 10017
(800) 777-3737 or (212) 685-4980, 4981, 4982

Glutathione is a unique sulfur-containing, naturally occurring amino acid composed of three component amino acids, called L-cysteine, L-glutamic acid, and glycine. Recently researchers have found that you can absorb the glutathione triple amino acids exceedingly fast when taken orally. The single product is best described as a free radical scavenger and oral chelating agent, which alters the action of dangerous peroxides. Glutathione preserves the health of your body by cleaning out its debris. It is a true chelator. A short discussion follows on the three amino acids making up the glutathione complex.

Cysteine is a sulfur-containing amino acid that displays definite chelating effects on excess copper by promoting its excretion, and thus is useful in rheumatoid arthritis. It protects cellular systems against the lethal effects of radiation exposure. L-Cysteine protects against acetaldehyde and acrolein in tobacco smoke and alcohol.

Glutamic acid (glutamine) sustains mental ability, improves brain metabolism, and works as a brain fuel in its amide form, which passes through the "blood-brain barrier."

Glycine (amino acetic acid) supplies a source of creatine for the treatment of muscular dystrophy. It improves blood circulation, gives a lift to the basal metabolism, and is known as an anti-hypoglycemic agent.

These chelating amino acids are available as food supplements from a few different distributors. Tyson & Associates Inc., 1661 Lincoln Boulevard, Suite 300, Santa Monica, California 90404; telephone inside California (213) 452-7844 or (800) 433-9750, outside California (800) 367-7744, supplies Aminoplex™, Aminoform™, Aminoplus™, and Aminohealth™, which are different types of amino acid formulae and individual free form amino acids to provide oral amino acid therapy. The Key Company, 734 North Harrison, Kirkwood, Missouri 63122; telephone (314) 965-6695 is a second amino acid supplement provider. The Ingler Company, 3330 S. Robertson Boulevard, Los Angeles, California 90034; telephone

(213) 378-2497, manufactures and distributes Aminessence™, a super amino acid of eighteen compounds in one product. Finally, a fourth supplier of amino acid supplements is the Dunsinane Company, 867 Queen Anne Road, Teaneck, New Jersey 07666; telephone (201) 836-9309.

Fiber is the part of food that is undigested by your body, such as apple skins, potato skins, wheat kernel husks, wheat bran, and other items that lend bulk but not necessarily nutrition to the diet. But fiber is a fine oral chelator for it grasps toxic agents from the intestinal tract and carries them out of the body in the stool. A low-fiber diet can give rise to heart disease, cancer of the colon and rectum, diverticulosis, varicose veins, phlebitis, and other degenerative diseases. Avoid these by self-chelating with fiber foods.

IV AND ORAL CHELATION THERAPY
RESTORE A POLICEMAN

Raymond Czarnecki, a 266-pound, 44-year-old police officer in Cicero, Illinois, had been experiencing a progressive loss of his exercise tolerance and a feeling of chest heaviness. Almost hourly he was taking Inderal, vasodilators, blood pressure pills, and diuretics. The poor fellow needed to drink tremendous amounts of liquids for his ever-present thirst, and people had been noting swelling about his eyes and ankles.

The policeman's constant feeling of fatigue and a sense that he could not continue doing his job brought officer Czarnecki to chelating physician Robert S. Waters, M.D., of Elmwood Park, Illinois, in May 1983. When he introduced himself to Dr. Waters, Raymond Czarnecki said, "Doc, I'm a candidate for the box. The way I've got it figured, I could check out any time. Both of my parents had heart trouble. I betcha I've got diabetes. (He did!) I'm so weak I can barely go to work. And because I feel so weak, I am not motivated to do anything about my condition like taking exercise or eating the proper diet. What I need is to get myself tuned up a little so that I can feel well enough to want to do something for myself."

Dr. Waters gave the patient a complete physical workup including glucose tolerance test, blood chemistry, blood count, thyroid profile, electrocardiogram, chest X-ray, a peripheral vascular non-invasive examination, continuous cardiac monitoring, hair mineral analysis, and more. Czarnecki's blood test readings were awful. His blood cholesterol level was too high at 305 mg % (mg % is the unit for measuring how much cholesterol is present in a specific percentage of blood taken), serum triglycerides shot up to 905 mg %, fasting blood sugar was 293, and the man's diabetic tolerance test had elevated his blood sugar to 372-348. His potassium was down to 3.3 and his chlorides were 90. The wreck's thickened blood could not be separated into its lipid components because it was so loaded with blood fats. The man's blood pressure was popping past 170/102. His peripheral vascular readings showed impairment of blood flow in his lower extremities and indicated that officer Czarnecki assuredly did feel intermittent claudication, which was one of his main complaints.

After only five chelation treatments his blood-sugar level came down to 107, his blood cholesterol dropped to 171 mg %, his blood triglycerides fell to 180 mg %, his potassium came up to 4.2, and his blood pressure remained consistently normal at 120/80. The man became healthy again. Dr. Waters was able to take Czarnecki off all medication. The patient reported that he was able to bound up two large flights of stairs without a stop, something he hadn't been able to do for nearly ten years. People told the policeman that he looked a dozen years younger since they had seen him last, just one month ago.

The patient now maintains his youthfulness with oral chelating agents including a full complement of the nutrients described in this chapter already and some of those discussed in Chapter Eleven. Dr. Waters prescribed them. The mineral imbalance that the policeman's hair analysis revealed is corrected completely. Police officer Raymond Czarnecki has become so happy with his results that he has formed a chapter of the Association for Cardiovascular Therapies in Cicero, Illinois. He wants everyone to feel the benefits of intravenous and oral chelation therapy as he has.

Nutritional Chelation Formulas and Their Sources

At age 49, Brunson Hollingsworth, a senior attorney in the law offices of Hollingsworth & Kramers of Hillsboro, Missouri, located about fifty miles south of St. Louis, Missouri, had a health history of increasingly severe chest pain. It so disabled him that he could no longer walk across the street from his office to attend hearings in the courthouse. Even worse, he was unable to engage in sexual intimacy with his wife, partly because of his physical disability and partly from his fear of bringing on a heart attack. Life was growing intolerable for the man. Although he did not verbalize the thought, it's possible that he felt life was not worth living in this incapacitated condition.

Mr. Hollingsworth had a cardiac catheterization (an angiogram) performed at the Barnes Hospital in St. Louis, on January 21, 1981. The angiologist reported that the patient suffered with a 4+ lesion (nearly the greatest amount of arterial blockage) in his distal right coronary artery and a 4+ lesion in the proximal left anterior descending coronary artery. According to the Barnes Hospital rating scale, 5+ is total arterial occlusion (a heart attack waiting to happen); 4+ is 75 percent to 99 percent occlusion (high grade blockage and almost always with symptoms); 3+ is 50 percent to 74 percent occlusion (may or may not experience symptoms); 2+ is 25 percent to 49 percent occlusion (seldom has symptoms); and 1+ is 1 percent to 24 percent occlusion (no symptoms, but most people have this degree of arterial clogging because of their lousy lifestyle).

Hollingsworth's cardiologist placed him on four heart disease drugs: Aldomet, Dyazide, Inderal, and Isordil. Coronary artery by-pass surgery was not recommended for the patient at that time, but the doctor said that it was an option he could fall back on later, if necessary.

The attorney went along with his symptoms, taking the heart remedies, and adjusting his activity from day to day in accordance with how he felt, starting from the moment he rose from bed in the morning. He was not managing well in his small town law practice. He perceived that he was not doing his share in the practice's workload and felt guilty and sad. An exercise stress test the man took indicated that he could walk the treadmill for only a very few minutes without feeling chest pain. Seeing this, the cardiologist reevaluated Hollingsworth and then strongly recommended a sec-ond arterial catheterization. The doctor's reconsideration also came out in favor of Hollingsworth having the coronary artery bypass operation. But the patient rejected his cardiologist's suggestions and took chelation therapy instead.

In October 1981, Hollingsworth went to visit Harvey Walker, Jr., M.D., Ph.D., of Clayton, Missouri, who is a member of the Ameri-can College of Advancement in Medicine. Dr. H. Walker performed the standard physical examination as directed by the ACAM proto-col and found that the patient was indeed a candidate for intrave-nous chelation treatment.

In an unusually short time, following only one IV infusion with EDTA, Hollingsworth reported a marked decrease in the amount and frequency of nitroglycerine he was forced to pop under his tongue each day. Angina was coming on less often. After just four chelation treatments the patient told how he was feeling better in every way. Ordinary movements and jobs that he had given up for fear of bringing on angina he found himself doing again. Sex no longer was a problem. He could rake leaves, take out the garbage, and stroll on an evening walk in the moonlight. One day he sat at his desk dictating legal briefs for two and a half hours without a break, more dictation than he had accomplished for the entire prior month.

Slowly Dr. H. Walker weaned the patient away from his cardiac drugs and no adverse effects developed. By December 4, the man was telling everyone in the chelation therapy clinic, such as fellow chelating patients, the staff members, and the physician, how improved his life had become. Now he was taking night court cases. His energy to do his share of the law practice work had returned, and he no longer was shunting off tasks onto his associates as he had to do earlier. He explained that in the winter of 1980, anginal pain had been so bad for him that his son was forced to start his car on cold mornings. With the completion of twelve chelation treatments, he was able to start the car himself without experiencing angina.

Hollingsworth has made the flat statement to all within earshot, "Anyone with my condition who isn't having chelation therapy is a damn fool."

By February 23, 1982, the patient had received twenty treatments. He reported that walking for two miles never brought on angina anymore, and his appetite for work, for exercise, and for frequent and vigorous sexual activity was strongly present. Limitations in these areas were what had motivated him to investigate chelation therapy in the first place. Hollingsworth said, "I am singing in the shower again. I haven't felt this good since before I was 40 years old, maybe even 35."

The attorney undertook an exercise treadmill test again on December 6, 1982, performed by the same cardiologist who had examined him before chelation therapy. Hollingsworth was able to walk five times longer than during the first test and his electrocardiogram showed much less heart ischemia existing than what had shown a year earlier. The cardiologist looked at these improvements and attributed them to "an act of God." He was unwilling to assign chelation therapy any credit for the better shape that Hollingsworth was in. The cardiologist said he would be convinced that the treatment had value only if he could see a repeat angiogram of the patient's coronary arteries. Not surprisingly, Hollingsworth, knowing that the angiographic procedure was connected with a .5 percent death rate on the table, was not about to put his life on the line just to make this narrow-minded establishment doctor a convert to chelation therapy.

The patient returned to Dr. Harvey Walker, Jr., for another series of booster treatments with EDTA and oral chelating agents. On October 5, 1983, he received his forty-third EDTA infusion. Hollingsworth takes his nutrient chelators as a sort of insurance policy against the return of any heart problem. His oral chelating nutritional supplements consist of the full vitamin B complex with vitamin C four times a day (Plus Products Formula Number 71), an additional 500 milligrams of vitamin C four times a day, vitamin E 400 IU four times a day, four capsules of lecithin 1,200 milligrams four times a day, the chelated minerals of chromium, zinc, magnesium, and selenium, and a multi-vitamin, multi-mineral pill (Basic Prevention™ made by Advanced Medical Nutrition Inc., of Hayward, California). The Basic Prevention™ formula and other oral chelating products made by Advanced Medical Nutrition Inc., will be described as this chapter's last series of entries.

Brunson Hollingsworth verbalizes poetically when he speaks or writes about the benefits he has experienced from taking chelation therapy and maintaining himself on the preventive oral chelation program. A letter he wrote to Dr. H. Walker, which I was privileged to read, indicates the man's uplifted attitude and "good to be alive" feeling. He is up at dawn, enjoys each day, works hard, plays harder, loves nature, and relishes his restoration to a fully active life.

ORAL CHELATING NUTRIENT FORMULAS

Non-invasive nutritional chelation therapy is treatment designed to remove the abnormal or metastatic deposits of calcium and other toxic elements from body cells. Metastatic calcium, as I have described in earlier chapters, may bring on pathological symptoms that are the first indications of degenerative disease. The products described in this and the next chapter, many by brand name or registered trademark, are just one part of an overall plan to improve blood circulation, increase blood vessel flexibility, improve organelle functioning, and in general bring the entire human organism back to homeostasis. Furthermore, of the various nutritional chelation formulas or chelating food substances about to be made known to you, some are available in health food stores, in pharmacies, directly from the manufacturer, or by multilevel marketing representatives. Others can only be gotten from a physician himself or may be purchased from the manufacturer directly, but with the stipulation that the product is being supplied by a doctor's prescription, which you must provide. Or, your physician can give verbal or written permission to the supplier that he or she may sell you the nutritional formula. Alternatively, some suppliers who sell their products to doctors have created separate consumer distribution companies or different brand names, often of the same exclusively distributed doctor product, for sale directly to the public. For a full disclosure of what the manufacturer provides, including questions as to package sizes, more detailed product descriptions, prices, quantities, discounts, and trade names not revealed here, contact the product maker using the information I am supplying.

Oral chelating agents are new, and a growing number of nutrient manufacturers are moving into the field. The oral chelators are usually designed for specific purposes. (1) They act as a stopgap for some patients who must interrupt their intravenous chelation therapy. (2) They are useful for people who cannot accept the invasive form of chelation treatment because of various medical reasons. (3) For those who have completed a course of infusions with EDTA, vitamin C, Eversol, or some other IV chelating solution, oral chelating agents may allow the people to stay on chelation therapy maintenance by utilizing daily dosages of the nutritional chelating products. (4) As a precursor to intravenous chelation treatment, oral chelating agents have helped the patient avoid any discomfort from sudden alteration of one's physiology by the invasive procedure. (5) Orally administered chelating nutrients and pharmaceuticals behave well as disease preventive measures against those many forms of cellular degenerations comprising physical, chemical, thermal, emotional, and mental stress in the body. If people living in industrialized Western societies were to apply the principles of preventive oral chelation therapy combined with the chelating benefits of aerobic exercise, it's likely that the incidence of heart and blood vessel diseases would be cut from 54.7 percent of all deaths each year to one quarter of that figure.

Of the formulas described in this chapter, a number of them contain naturally chelating food substances not yet described, such as mucopolysaccharides, N,N-dimethylglycine, bromelain, lecithin, and others. Most of these undescribed supplemental nutrients, including orally administered chelating pharmaceuticals, will be briefly discussed in Chapter Twelve.

First, be advised again that your daily performance of aerobic exercise is an important technique for self-administered chelation therapy. George M. Miller, of Scottsdale, Arizona, advocates that exercise is as necessary to self-chelation as are all the other nutritional ingredients suggested here. Mr. Miller warns: "Without exercise the non-invasive mineral chelation technique will not be long-lasting. Walking is the exercise of choice. Walking can improve poor circulation, heal a sick heart and make one healthier and happier. The most important ingredient in regard to walking is to walk every day."

Miller goes on to give some friendly advice about the technique of walking, if you aren't in the habit of taking daily exercise. He says, "Start slowly, maybe 15 minutes each day. After a couple of weeks, increase the time to 30 minutes each day, and increase the pace. Two weeks later increase walking time to 45 minutes and then to one hour. As your stamina increases you will be able to walk three to four miles each hour. Walking calms the nerves, increases circulation and lowers blood pressure. It has been said by some, 'The roadway back to good health is long and difficult.' Well let's get on that roadway and start walking, today and every day."

Garry F. Gordon, M.D., my medical consultant for *The Chelation Answer*, has created an oral chelation therapy formula called Added Protection III™. It provides the chelating and nutritional benefits of two amino acids (cysteine and methionine) plus thirty vitamins and minerals, three different forms of magnesium for tissue-specific bioactivity, and beta-carotene. This formula is sold only to licensed health professionals for dispensing to patients; however, if you are looking for a nutritionist, physician, chiropractor, or another doctor who treats disease with nutrition and/or chelation therapy, the manufacturing company invites you to use its toll-free telephone number for a health professional referral in your area. Please see page 214 for further information on the manufacturer, Advanced Medical Nutrition Inc.

The Advanced Medical Nutrition product, Added Protection III™, is a high-potency, hypoallergenic, vitamin-mineral chelating formula. It comes in bottles of 180 tablets, each bottle containing a thirty-day supply. It is formulated with or without copper, which is included depending on the patient's individual hair mineral analysis. His or her holistic physician reads the hair analysis report that is returned by Advanced Medical Nutrition and then determines whether the patient should receive the formula containing copper.

Six tablets of Added Protection III™ contain the following ingredients and dosages:

Vitamin A (Palmitate)	10,000 IU
Beta-carotene	5,000 IU
Vitamin D-3	200 IU
Vitamin E (d-alpha tocopheryl succinate)	400 IU
Vitamin C	1,200 mg
Vitamin B-1	100 mg
Vitamin B-2	50 mg
Niacin	40 mg
Niacinamide	150 mg
Pantothenic acid (d-calcium pantothenate)	500 mg
Vitamin B-6	100 mg
Vitamin B-12	100 mcg
Folic acid	800 mcg
Biotin	300 mcg
Choline bitartrate	150 mg
Inositol	100 mg
Citrus bioflavonoid complex	100 mg
PABA (para-amino-benzoic acid)	50 mg
Calcium	500 mg
Magnesium ascorbate	166 mg
Magnesium aspartate	183 mg
Magnesium oxide	151 mg
Potassium aspartate	99 mg
Iron fumarate	20 mg
Zinc aspartate	30 mg
Copper aspartate	2 mg
Manganese aspartate	20 mg
Iodine (kelp)	200 mcg
Chromium (glucose tolerance component)	200 mcg
Selenium	200 mcg

Molybdenum	100 mcg
Trace elements from sea vegetation	100 mg
L-Cysteine	250 mg
DL-Methionine	62.5 mg

Among the best of the consumer-available, multilevel marketed oral chelating nutrients are the Golden Pride *Formulas for Health*—in particular Golden Pride Formula I. This liquid-based nutritional supplement contains ingredients that provide a near-equivalent effect of intravenous chelation therapy (except that the orally administered form does not work as fast). For instance, Golden Pride Formula I uses honey to carry nutritional components orally. The chelated formula uses EDTA or its equivalent for its chelation effect. Then, simulating chelation therapy's intravenous infuser mechanism is bee pollen.

In each Golden Pride *Formulas for Health* Formula I product jar, there is 8,000 milligrams of royal jelly, which contains pantothenic acid (vitamin B-5), pyridoxine (vitamin B-6), cobalamin (vitamin B-12), ascorbic acid (vitamin C), and magnesium chloride. Also, the royal jelly is a highly concentrated source of acetylcholine (the brain vitamin).

It is suggested that people take from one to four teaspoons of the product each day. Users of the product (over 1,000 letters of praise have been received by the company) reported dramatic benefits among which angina pectoris was completely eliminated, bypass operations became unnecessary in remarkable instances, diabetic retinopathy disappeared in three cases, arthritic symptoms were relieved, and many more conditions improved. Most of all, the product is amazingly effective for cardiovascular health.

For more information about the nutritional quality of Golden Pride *Formulas for Health* Formula I, or to learn about distributing it, write or telephone the headquarters offices of Golden Pride Inc., where you will find the company president Harry Hersey, 1501 North Point Parkway, West Palm Beach, Florida 33407; telephone (305) 586-7778. Or contact Regional Director Pat Lawson, a key distribution executive in the Golden Pride Inc. multilevel marketing downline organization, 3493 Augusta Drive, Ijamsville, Maryland 21754; toll-free telephone (800) 233-6550; Maryland residents: (301) 831-6005.

A number of manufacturers and distributors offer oral chelating and intravenous chelating products primarily through physicians' offices or through pharmacies by prescription. Contact the following companies either for information about how to acquire their oral chelating products or for referrals to physicians in your area who are using oral chelators or intravenous chelation therapy.

Phyne Pharmaceuticals Inc. and American Pharmaceutical Enterprises Inc., both companies under the presidency of James Critchlow, Ph.D., offer pharmaceuticals for chelation therapy and preventive medicine as well as dimethyl sulfoxide creams and liquids. Dr. Critchlow and his two companies are located at 5121 Southwest 90th Avenue, Cooper City, Florida 33328; telephone (305) 434-7106.

Thorne Research Inc., Al Czap, president, offers a complete line of nutritional supplements, in two-piece hard gelatin capsules, designed for the chemically sensitive patient and available exclusively through physicians and by prescription in selected pharmacies. Thorne Research Inc. is located at 610 Andover Park East, Seattle, Washington 98188; telephone (206) 575-0777.

Miller Pharmacal Group Inc. provides a wide range of minerals, vitamins, amino acids, injectables and related products, and trace mineral analysis. Miller Pharmacal Group Inc. is found at 245 West Roosevelt Road, West Chicago, Illinois 60185; telephone (312) 231-3632 and outside Illinois (800) 323-2935. John Wonsil, Miller Pharmacal's vice president of sales, is happy to provide any medical consumer with a referral to a nearby physician who is skilled in administering chelation therapy.

Metagenics Inc. offers nutritional supplements based on scientifically validated nutritional formulations including vitamins, minerals, amino acids, and others. Contact Metagenics Inc. at 23180 Del Lago, Laguna Hills, California 92653; telephone (714) 855-1718.

The McGuff Company produces all products necessary for intravenous EDTA chelation therapy including: small and large volume parenteral drugs, IV flow control products, oral nutritional support products, and a host of related items for the physician. The company's main nutritional support product used by chelating physicians for their patients is called "qf." For information and physician referrals, you may get in touch with Scott Nixon, national sales manager for the McGuff Company, at 3625 West MacArthur Boulevard, #306,

Santa Ana, California 92704; telephone (714) 545-2491 or (800) 367-6644 or outside California (800) 854-7220.

GY and N Nutriment Pharmacology Inc. offers products and supplies for chelation therapy, injectable vitamins, minerals, and IV solutions. The company also offers a complete line of oral vitamins, minerals, glandulars, and special-use oral products. Its laboratory services include hair, plasma, urine, red blood cells, and whole blood minerals and amino acid analyses from urine or plasma. You may contact company co-owners Gil McGrath and Bob Woods at GY and N Nutriment Pharmacology Inc., P. O. Box 2252, Carlsbad, California 92008; telephone in California (805) 522-6699 or (800) 526-3030 or outside California (800) 445-2122.

Douglas Laboratories, a Division of HVL Inc. offers over 250 nutritional supplements sold only to physicians. They include amino acids, digestive enzymes, glandulars, lipotropics, minerals/multi-minerals, multiple vitamin and mineral formulas, homeopathic formulas, and more. For doctor referrals or information about the company's major nutritional support oral agent, Ultra Preventive III, which is utilized by chelating physicians, contact Jeff Lioon, president of Douglas Laboratories, at P. O. Box 8583, Wabash & Main, Pittsburgh, Pennsylvania 15220; telephone (412) 937-0122 or toll-free in Pennsylvania (800) 542-1400 or outside Pennsylvania (800) 245-4440.

Dove Medical Supplies features a complete line of disposable medical products, injectable drugs, dialysis supplies and solutions. Find Dove Medical Supplies at 315 Grand Boulevard, Vancouver, Washington 98661; (206) 694-9405.

Cell Life International offers a complete line of multi-vitamins, benzaldehyde E, and trace mineral products in tablet and powder form. Reach Cell Life International at 9373 Activity Road, Unit I, San Diego, California 92126; telephone (619) 271-7613.

Bio-Tech offers (1) single-entity and combination oral and injectable products for the preventive medicine physician, such as chelated minerals, essential fatty acids, digestives, amino acids, bromelain; (2) mineral analysis; and (3) guidance programs for the new, as well as experienced, chelating doctor. Get in touch with Bio-Tech at P. O. Box 1992, Fayetteville, Arkansas 72702; telephone (501) 443-9148.

Bio-Therapeutics provides a complete line of nutritional vitamin supplements and plant extracts. Find Bio-Therapeutics at P. O. Box 1348, Green Bay, Wisconsin 54305; telephone (414) 435-4200 or outside Wisconsin (800) 553-2370.

Biomed Foods provides a full line of whole food antioxidant enzyme complexes that quench free radical formation and produce a type of oral chelation effect. Get in touch with Biomed Foods at 2639 South King Street, Suite 206, Honolulu, Hawaii 96826; telephone (800) 468-7578. Biomed has a consumer line of enzymes sold in health food stores and by mail order. The company's California office is maintained by Zane Baranowski who gives assistance and product information at 597 Glenwood Cut-Off, Scotts Valley, California 95066-2601; telephone (800) 331-5888.

Biotics Research Corporation offers food supplements such as enzymes, minerals, vitamins, superoxide dismutase, coenzyme Q_{10}, octacosanol, porphyrine, emulsions, neonatal glandulars, and amino acids. For physician referrals or product information, the company president, Dennis Deluca, may be reached at Biotics Research Corporation, P. O. Box 36888, Houston, Texas 77236; telephone (713) 240-8010 or (800) 231-5777.

Klaire Laboratories Inc. offers nutritional supplements catering to the highly sensitive individual. It also offers a full line of cardiovascular nutrients and microorganism formulations such as *Lactobacillus acidophilus*. You may reach Klaire Laboratories Inc. at 1573 West Seminole Street, San Marcos, California 92069; telephone (619) 744-9680.

Robar Pharmaceuticals Inc. features a complete line of injectables, tablets, and capsules for the physician practicing preventive medicine. Contact Robar Pharmaceuticals Inc. at 1630 Falcon, Suite 106, Desoto, Texas 75115; telephone (214) 224-9640.

Bob's Discount Drugs Inc. provides many supplements and nutritional products for the environmentally and chemically sensitive patient. Stocked at all times are starch-, yeast-, and sugar-free vitamins. Find Bob's Discount Drugs Inc. at 2800 South 18th Street, Birmingham, Alabama 35209; telephone (205) 879-6551 or toll-free (800) 227-2627.

Health Values Corporation features regenerative herbal formulas, mineral transport systems, and pharmaceutical amino acids in a physician's health-enhancement program. Learn about Health Values Corporation products at 430 North State College, Anaheim, California 92806; telephone (714) 772-5854.

Karuna Corporation presents a complete line of nutritional supplements such as MaxEPA, MAXXUM, SGP, herbal-vitamin, mineral combinations, and homeopathics. Find out more by contacting Karuna Corporation, 200 Gate Five Road, Suite 102, Sausalito, California 94965; telephone (415) 331-5097.

Allergy Research Group and Nutricology Inc., both functioning from the same offices, offer hypoallergenic vitamin and mineral supplements, research literature, and technical and medical consumer books. Under the direction of Stephen Levine, Ph.D., the two companies have introduced important original nutritional products. Leading original products include non-corn-buffered vitamin C, Anti-Ox, organic germanium, and Oxysport Pe9+ Egg Lecithin for Acquired Immune Deficiency Syndrome (AIDS). Allergy Research Group and Nutricology Inc. is located at 400 Preda Street, P. O. Box 489, San Leandro, California 94577-0489; telephone (415) 639-4572 or toll-free (800) 545-9960.

Vitaline Formulas manufactures medical nutritional formulas such as Che-detox, an oral detoxification formula, organic germanium, coenzyme Q_{10}, natural lipotropic formulas, bromelain, superoxide dismutase, pyridoxine/alpha-ketoglutarate complex, and high lipase pancreatin. Vitaline offers its nutritional supplements to physicians, hospitals, pharmacies, and other licensed health care professionals. Contact Vitaline Formulas at P. O. Box 6757, Incline Village, Nevada 89450; telephone toll-free (800) 648-4755.

Barry Vishny, M.D., medical director of the La Paz Preventive Health Care Foundation in Mission Viejo, California, utilizes therapeutic oral chelating agents but not intravenous chelation injections as part of his integrated approach to medical care. He considers oral chelation therapy combined with an appropriate chelation diet part of the natural treatment modalities to which he is committed. Dr. Vishny furnished me with a number of case histories in which he employed a highly effective oral chelator called Angio Guard™ for his cardiovascular patients. In Dr. Vishny's practice, Angio Guard™ proved quite successful for the relief and/or reversal of ischemic heart disease with episodes of fainting, diabetes, diabetic retinopathy, atherosclerosis, bilateral stasis dermatitis in both legs, poor vision, high blood pressure, and arthritis.

Angio Guard™ is manufactured and distributed exclusively for dispensing to patients by their physicians. The producer is an organization of health care practitioners dedicated to the promotion of good health. The organization has the name NF Physicians Formula Inc., Dr. Bruce Canvasser, President, and Jonathan Means, National Sales Director, 3388 Southeast 20th, Portland, Oregon 97202; telephone (503) 232-5710 or toll-free inside Oregon at (800) 325-9326 or outside Oregon at (800) 547-4891.

As mentioned, NF Angio Guard™ is a comprehensive nutritional program geared to the needs of the holistic physician for his or her cardiovascular patient in the preventive maintenance of the heart and circulatory system. It provides a full complement of nutritional and botanical factors known to aid in the restoration and stabilization of circulatory homeostasis. Designed by medical professionals for clinical application, this product provides the patient and physician with a simple yet scientific means of natural restorative treatment in the management of degenerative diseases involving the heart and circulatory system. It is an adjunctive source of high quality nutrients and safe, harmless botanical medicines.

The ingredients in three capsules of Angio Guard™ consist of:

Potassium (aspartate)	99 mg
Magnesium (aspartate)	50 mg
L-Cysteine	200 mg
Taurine	150 mg
Crataegus (hawthorn)	500 mg
Ginkgo biloba	100 mg
Taraxacum	100 mg
Uva ursi	100 mg
Equisetum	100 mg
Ascorbic acid	100 mg
Niacin	100 mg
Dimethylglycine	100 mg
L-Carnitine	150 mg
Pyridoxyl-5 phosphate	25 mg
Chondroitin sulphate-4	100 mg

For full information including price schedules, quantity purchasing, and a list of doctors using the product, contact NF Physicians Formula Inc., the manufacturer of Angio Guard™, through the company's sales director, Jonathan Means.

Mankind's concepts of nutrition have changed with the advent of chelation therapy. In seeking to increase the human life expectancy and the degree of health, some investigators have developed injectables and oral nutrient chelating formulas that contain synergistic ingredients. The injectables are used by physicians to bring about controlled therapeutic effects for sick patients. But these nutrients are all different. They spark one's imagination concerning their properties and how they might benefit individuals in both a therapeutic and a disease preventive manner. One manufacturer of injectables and specific nutrient substances dispensed by doctors, Merit Pharmaceuticals, has investigated symbiotic properties and come up with two different orally administered chelating formulas. In the past, these formulations have been provided to patients only through physicians' offices and clinics. Now the president of Merit Pharmaceuticals, Chuck Farha, is allowing consumers to purchase directly from the company so as to be able to sell the company's oral chelating products to the public.

To acquire products similar to those that you could formerly get only from your physician, go right to Chuck Farha's newly established marketing arm at Merit Pharmaceuticals. Telephone or write to Merit Pharmaceuticals at 2611 San Fernando Road, Los Angeles, California 90065; telephone (213) 227-4258, call toll-free outside California (800) 421-9657 or toll-free inside California (800) 252-8223 for price schedules on the two oral chelating products; one is called Ecolovit™ and the other has the name M/CHE Pro™. Both formulas from Fern Laboratories come packaged in bottles of 180 tablets. Moreover, the daily dosage for these two formulas is the same, six tablets each day in evenly divided doses as a prevention against getting cardiovascular disease and/or three tablets daily as maintenance care after you have gone through a course of intravenous chelation therapy.

Each Ecolovit™ nutritionally formulated tablet contains the following ingredients and dosages:

Niacinamide	33.33 mg
Ascorbic acid	33.33 mg
PABA	2.50 mg
Inositol	16.66 mg
Rutin (bioflavonoid)	4.16 mg
Citrus bioflavonoids	16.66 mg
Calcium (dicalcium phosphate)	25.00 mg
Phosphorus	12.5 mg
Calcium gluconate	8.33 mg
Betaine	4.16 mg
Glutamic acid	16.66 mg
Lysine	4.16 mg
Methionine	8.33 mg
Bile salts	1.66 mg
Papain	1.66 mg
Dried milk	4.58 mg
Organ meat	4.58 mg
Soy protein	4.58 mg
Yeast	4.58 mg
Pineapple concentrate	0.83 mg
Vitamin A (acetate)	833.33 mg
Vitamin D	66.66 mg
Vitamin B-12	16.66 mcg
Vitamin E (d-alpha succinate)	16.66 IU
Folic acid	0.016 mg
Biotin	4.16 mg
Choline bitartrate	25.00 mg
Iodine (kelp)	0.0125 mg
Pancreatin N.F.	4.16 mg
Iron	1.66 mg
Copper	0.33 mg
Manganese	0.83 mg
Magnesium	41.66 mg
Zinc	2.50 mg
Chromium	0.016 mg

Molybdenum	0.016 mg
Potassium	12.50 mg
Thiamin	4.16 mg
Riboflavin	1.66 mg
Pyridoxine	8.33 mg

Produced in a base containing rose hips powder and acerola, this Ecolovit™ formula is free of wax, sugar, starch, and artificial coloring. The Ecolovit™ tablet's minerals are chelated with hydrolyzed protein for more complete absorption in the gut.

Fern Laboratories also makes available chelated minerals combined in one M/CHE Pro™ tablet with essential and non-essential amino acids. An essential amino acid is one that is absolutely necessary for normal growth and development but cannot be synthesized by the body. Essential amino acids are usually obtained from protein-rich foods in the diet, such as liver, eggs, and dairy products. If you are following the macrobiotic diet or the Pritikin diet, have allergies to such protein-rich foods, or for some other reason find an inadequate amount of the eight essential amino acids in what you consume, M/CHE Pro™ is an appropriate formulation for you to add to your daily routine of nourishment. The essential amino acids are tryptophan, lysine, phenylalanine, threonine, valine, methionine, leucine, and isoleucine, all of which (and more) are found in M/CHE Pro™. Six tablets of M/CHE Pro™ contain:

Protein	1.62 g
Iodine	0.15 mcg
Iron	10.00 mg
Magnesium	30.00 mg
Copper	1.00 mg
Zinc	2.00 mg
Manganese	2.00 mg
Potassium	20.00 mg

Six tablets of M/CHE Pro™ will also provide the following amino acids:

Alanine	68 mg
Arginine	74 mg
Aspartic acid	179 mg
Glutamic acid	226 mg
Glycine	107 mg
Histidine	45 mg
Isoleucine	101 mg
Cystine	16 mg
Hydroxyproline	37 mg
Leucine	136 mg
Lysine	425 mg
Methionine	110 mg
Phenylalanine	103 mg
Proline	39 mg
Threonine	84 mg
Serine	115 mg
Tryptophan	27 mg
Tyrosine	74 mg
Valine	117 mg

With cardiovascular disease ranking number one in mortality and morbidity throughout the United States and other Western countries, numerous nutritional aspects of hardening of the arteries have been named. Diet can be a factor in hardening of the arteries; you also may be deficient in or require more amino acids, endocrine substances, minerals, and vitamins than the average person for your cardiovascular system to function well. The scientific literature supports the rational use of individual amino acids, especially cysteine, although it is not one of the essentials that I previously cited. Cysteine is among the many ingredients in an orally administered chelating formula called Eze-Flow™, produced by Vega Laboratories, under the direction of the company's president Jeremiah deMichaelis.

Vega Laboratories, headquartered at 2800 South Main Street, Suite A, Santa Ana, California 92707; telephone (714) 250-0532, is a person-to-person multilevel marketing organization. It makes and then sells Eze-Flow™ directly to the public through a distribution network of trained laypersons and doctors who are vitally interested in cardiovascular health, full body health, avoidance of degenerative diseases, and the holistic concept of living. The multilevel marketing network actually consists of just ordinary people who usually swallow their own chelating product every day. These distributors look the picture of optimal health. They provide their oral chelating agents to others whom they know, care about, and believe will benefit from the disease prevention program or other therapeutic aspects of taking somewhat higher doses of vital nutritional supplements, as embodied in the Eze-Flow™ formula.

The formula furnishes minerals in a highly assimilable form for purposes of lowering serum cholesterol by activating cholesterol esterases in the blood vessel walls. Eze-Flow™ minerals such as selenium, manganese, magnesium, zinc, chromium, and potassium aid in the elimination of excess calcium from the tissues, benefit and improve memory and concentration, promote deep and restful sleep, and generally act much like the new generation of calcium channel blocker drugs, but without the side effects, and in a physiologically acceptable way. They permit no cellular accumulation of sodium and calcium.

The other ingredients in Eze-Flow™ such as the full complement of B-complex vitamins, and vitamins A, D, C, and E plus raw glandular extracts, aid in the delivery of oxygen to the tissues, help lower serum fats, prevent too much lactic acid buildup, improve heart functioning, and increase energy.

Can something so nutritive and safe as these Eze-Flow™ food supplementing ingredients improve the quality of life? Yes! Knowledgeable nutritional scientists, as represented by the holistic physicians belonging to the International Academy of Preventive Medicine and the Academy of Orthomolecular Medicine, believe that such a nutrient formula can do so. The sort of ingredients included in Eze-Flow™ are prescribed by the doctors.

Vega Laboratories' scientists suggest that eight tablets of Eze-Flow™ be taken each day, in divided doses of four in the morning and four in the evening. They recommend that you pop this amount in your mouth with each of two meals for at least three months, after which you can cut the dose to just four tablets per day for three months. A maintenance level is then reached of one or two tablets per day for continued oral chelating mechanisms ongoing in your body. You will thus retain an elevated blood titer of nutrient protection against free radicals that are implicated in degenerative processes. The product comes packaged in bottles of 120 tablets.

For full information about how you may become an Eze-Flow™ distributor or for a referral to your nearest distributor for acquiring the product for personal use, contact Jeremiah deMichaelis at the Vega Laboratories address that I gave earlier in this report.

Eight tablets of the Eze-Flow™ oral chelation formula contain the following ingredients and dosages:

Vitamin A (fish liver oil)	40,000 IU
Vitamin D (fish liver oil)	800 IU
Vitamin E (d-alpha tocopherol)	650 IU
Vitamin C (vegetable source)	4,500 mg
Vitamin B-1	200 mg
Vitamin B-2	20 mg
Vitamin B-6	170 mg
Vitamin B-12	165 mcg
Niacin	80 mg
Niacinamide	20 mg
Pantothenic acid (cal-panto & yeast)	350 mg
PABA (para-amino-benzoic acid)	380 mg
Choline bitartrate	725 mg
Inositol	40 mg
Folic acid	400 mcg
Biotin	100 mcg
Calcium (dicalcium phosphate & oyster shell)	600 mg
Magnesium (oxide)	300 mg
Potassium (chloride)	99 mg
Iron (fumarate)	10 mg
Iodine (potassium iodide & kelp)	125 mcg
Copper	250 mcg
Chromium (yeast)	100 mcg
Manganese	5 mg
Zinc	28 mg

Selenium (yeast)	250 mcg
Cysteine hydrochloride	750 mg
Methionine	200 mg
Adrenal substance	50 mg
Thymus substance	100 mg

The oral chelation technique is a means to stop the clock on premature aging. Biologic aging actually starts in early fetal life. Calcium deposits increase in the body; magnesium steadily decreases, and this effect is more noticeable in middle and old age. Non-invasive chelation therapy that is being delineated in this second part of *The Chelation Way: The Complete Book of Chelation Therapy* is not a cure for all bodily ills and is not as effective as the intravenous variety of chelation therapy. But it is a specific treatment program aimed at reducing pathological changes through the removal of abnormal deposits of calcium. Such metastatic calcium depositions have been known to cause a disease state.

Another advanced nutrient manufacturer and supplier has perfected a formulation for oral chelation therapy. Lanpar Company, a division of American Bio-Search, 7101 Carpenter Freeway, Dallas, Texas 75247; telephone toll-free (800) 527-9425 or (214) 630-8484 has created Ascorbopath™ therapy, a comprehensive nutritional plan to improve blood circulation.

Ascorbopath™ comes in case lots of twenty-eight vials and is dispensed to patients by their physicians. It is a carefully formulated ascorbated mineral supplement forming the base for the non-invasive chelation therapy technique. This orally administered technique is accomplished by the large ascorbate intake, which increases the urinary excretion of several body minerals. Calcium and magnesium are mainly affected. The ascorbate chelation of calcium is of prime importance using this procedure since there is potential benefit of removing calcium not deposited under good physiological conditions. To avoid mineral loss that would be deemed undesirable in this chelation process and, in fact, to enhance the chelation procedure, added ascorbated minerals insure that adequate levels are present in the body. The ascorbated minerals used in the Lanpar Company formula are partially chelated and partially electrostatically associated.

Up to one vial of Ascorbopath™ is the daily dosage. The product usually is started slowly and raised by milliliters (or micrograms), as tolerated by the patient. Ascorbopath™ can be mixed with any convenient liquid. If the dose is raised slowly, the patient's bowel tolerance for the high amount of vitamin C can be improved.

Each vial of Ascorbopath™ contains the following ingredients and dosages:

Ascorbic acid	2,000 mg
Sodium ascorbate	865 mg
Magnesium ascorbate	2,323 mg
Zinc ascorbate	64 mg
Manganese ascorbate	30 mg
Selenium ascorbate	27 mcg
Potassium aspartate	103 mg
Magnesium aspartate	105 mg
Potassium citrate	161 mg

This Ascorbopath™ non-invasive chelation therapy technique recommended by Lanpar Company is utilized by M. Paul Dommers, M.D., of Belvidere, Illinois. Dr. Dommers makes the following suggestions to his patients about how to use the product:

This box will last you approximately one month. Mix Ascorbopath™ with any liquid (for drinking). Dosage:

Day 1. Take the equivalent of one line marked on the vial.

Day 2. Take the equivalent of two lines marked on the vial.

Day 3. Take the equivalent of three lines marked on the vial.

Day 4. Take the equivalent of four lines marked on the vial.

Day 5. Take the equivalent of five lines marked on the vial.

Day 6 and Thereafter. Take half of the vial in the morning and half the vial in the evening; a total of one vial per day.

If diarrhea occurs, reduce the dosage to half a vial per day.

Adjunctive to the Ascorbopath™ program, Lanpar Company also furnishes pure granulated and unbleached lecithin in fourteen-ounce jars, which Dr. Dommers tells his patients to use in the following manner:

Day 1. Take half a level tablespoonful mixed in liquid or food.

Day 2. Take one level tablespoonful mixed in liquid or food.

Day 3. Take two level tablespoonfuls mixed in liquid or food.

Day 4. Take four level tablespoonfuls mixed in liquid or food.

Day 5. Take four to six level tablespoonfuls mixed in liquid or food, depending on your bowel tolerance. If diarrhea occurs, reduce your dosage.

Combined with these Ascorbopath™ and lecithin ingredients, the Lanpar Company oral chelation technique makes use of magnesium orotate 500 mg and magnesium 33 mg in an enteric film-coated tablet called Mag-Plus™ (bottles of 100 tablets), bromelain 105 mg and inositol gluconate 61.4 mg and N, N-dimethylglycine hydrochloride 38.6 mg in a product called DMG™ (bottles of 60 tablets), natural d-alpha tocopheryl acetate 400 IU in a product called Vitamin E™ (bottles of 100 capsules), and niacin or nicotonic acid time release 500 mg in a product called Niacin TR-500™ (bottles of 100 tablets).

Dr. Dommers' patient instructions for each of these additions to his oral chelating program are:

1. Take one Mag-Plus™ tablet in the morning and one tablet at night.
2. Take one Bromotol™ tablet by buccal administration (between your cheek and gum) three times a day.
3. Take one tablet of DMG™ four times a day.
4. Take one tablet of Vitamin E™ three times a day.
5. Start with one tablet of Niacin TR-500™ each day. If severe flushing or faintness occurs, reduce to half a tablet a day.

Based on fifteen years of research and manufacturing nutritional supplements for dispensing by holistic physicians, Alfred "Fred" Rechberger, president of Biometabolic Laboratories of Manchester, New Hampshire, decided to make and distribute oral chelating agents directly to the public. Mr. Rechberger assigned his other company, Essential Organics, Organic Park, P. O. Box 325, Derry, New Hampshire 03038; telephone (603) 432-5022, the task of creating an oral chelating formula for public distribution. Essential Organics came up with an exceedingly complete formulation called Oralkel™.

Oralkel™ is packaged in bottles of 180, 360, and 540 tablets as a dietary supplement for oral chelation therapy. The standard dosage is two or three tablets to be taken with meals morning, noon, and evening. The product can be acquired by contacting the Essential Organics Company. Oralkel™ is derived from natural sources such as fish oil extracts, super high potency yeast, rose hips concentrate, vegetable oil extract, bone meal, kelp, sea water, and other natural sources. Nothing is synthetically produced.

Nine tablets of Oralkel™ supply the following ingredients and dosages:

Vitamin A & beta-carotene (pro-vitamin A)	25,000 IU
Vitamin D	800 IU
Vitamin E	400 IU
Vitamin C	4,000 mg
Vitamin B-1	50 mg
Vitamin B-2	50 mg
Vitamin B-6	100 mg
Vitamin B-12	150 mcg
Niacinamide & niacin	200 mg
Pantothenic acid	150 mcg
Biotin	60 mcg
Calcium (chelated)	400 mg
Magnesium (chelated)	250 mg
Iron (chelated)	18 mg
Iodine (kelp)	225 mcg
Copper (chelated)	250 mcg
Chromium (GTF, chelated)	200 mcg
Manganese (chelated)	5 mg

Potassium (chelated)	99 mg
Selenium (proteinate)	100 mcg
Zinc (chelated)	30 mg
Mineral complex (containing 60 trace minerals)	100 mg
Choline bitartrate	750 mg
Inositol	50 mg
Para-amino-benzoic acid	100 mg
Cysteine hydrochloride	750 mg
Methionine	250 mg
Adrenal, pituitary, thymus complex	150 mg
Superoxide dismutase, catalase, peroxidase complex	20 mg
Alginate, lecithin, pectin complex	250 mg
Rose hips, bioflavonoids, hesperidin, rutin	250 mg

A growing company run by a dynamic scientist with an abiding interest in oral chelation therapy offers a complete line of nutritional supplements specifically designed to accomplish the cellular process for removing toxic elements and replacing them with metabolic support. Jonathan Rothschild is president of Cardiovascular Research Ltd., and can be reached at 1061 Shary Circle, Concord, California 94518; telephone (415) 827-2636 or (415) 827-3322 or toll-free outside California at (800) 351-9429. The two main oral chelators manufactured by Cardiovascular Research Ltd. are mucopolysaccharide concentrate and carnitine (vitamine B-T).

Mucopolysaccharide concentrate is a nutrient containing the complete spectrum of essential mucopolysaccharides in a concentrated form, including chondroitin sulfates, heparin, and hyaluronic acid. These carefully extracted substances have been shown to clear lipids and to retard the arteriosclerotic and aging processes within the arterial walls. (In Chapter Twelve, more information on mucopolysaccharides is included.)

The Cardiovascular Research product has been used by prominent physicians and researchers in academic medicine and is considered a highly potent oral chelating agent. Some of the clinical benefits observed following its use include reduction in angina pectoris, improvement in blood plasma parameters, better blood levels for normal total serum cholesterol and triglycerides as well as improved liver function studies. A complete bibliography is available upon your requesting it from Jonathan Rothschild.

The ingredients contained in each mucopolysaccharide-concentrate capsule compose a specifically prepared fraction of 300 milligrams of acid mucopolysaccharides derived from bovine connective tissue. Suggested usage is to take three capsules daily, or as directed by a physician. The mucopolysaccharides are precipitated from these cartilaginous extracts through papain hydrolysis under laboratory-controlled conditions. They have been assayed for biological potency and anti-thrombic activity by independent researchers.

Carnitine (vitamin B-T) is a naturally occurring amine found in all living tissue, with the highest concentrations present in the adrenal glands and cardiac muscle.

Researchers have recently found that carnitine is an effective nutritional agent in managing ischemic heart disease, cardiac arrhythmias, and elevated triglyceride levels. Moreover this safe and effective nutrient raises serum HDL levels. (An HDL is a high-density lipoprotein, the beneficial component of the cholesterol molecule.) This serum elevation is especially important in patients who are unable to exercise.

The anti-fatigue effects of carnitine have also been observed in healthy individuals following prolonged muscle effort, and it is used by athletes in endurance sports.

According to numerous published studies, a minimum daily dose of 900 milligrams of carnitine is required in order for therapeutic benefit to be derived. However, this nutrient works rapidly and triglyceride levels drop to within normal limits in fifteen days among 73 percent of patients studied.

Each capsule of the Cardiovascular Research carnitine product contains 550 milligrams of D,L carnitine in the 100 percent pure, crystalline form. Suggested usage is to take two capsules a day, or as directed by a physician.

Kurt W. Donsbach, Ph.D., of Rosarito Beach, Baja, California, Mexico, of Hospital Santa Monica, is the inventive nutritional genius who first developed the concept of oral chelating agents for sale directly to the medical consumer. He joined with Keith Kenyon, M.D., of Glendale, California to create Orachel™. The ingredients combined in Orachel™ were formulated in two years. They have the properties of assisting the circulatory system, with practically no side effects involved except as might be present with any nutrient substance taken into the body. Dr. Donsbach does warn of such side effects as flatulence, indigestion, fatigue, or nausea. In fact, mild discomforts could materialize for any of the oral chelating agents described in this text.

Flatulence comes from a change in the intestinal flora resulting in taking potent nutrients. Lower bowel gas may occur for a few days and be over within a week.

Indigestion could come on from not taking the oral chelating agents with meals. A meal containing some animal or vegetable protein is best. It isn't advisable to take oral chelation therapy on an empty stomach.

Fatigue may be present because the oral chelators can bring about a considerable release of debris into the blood stream with a temporary decrease in the body's ability to carry oxygen. This could produce a need to have more rest and relaxation for perhaps a week. The side effect of fatigue probably happens most often to people who require oral chelation therapy the most.

Nausea could result from any intolerance by the body to one or more of the food supplements. People allergic to yeast, for instance, may not respond well to B-complex vitamins or selenium derived from yeast. Many sources of B vitamins exist. In the case of selenium, the type of selenium made from oceanic sources should be used instead.

Such minor side effects might occur in as many as 5 percent of everyone who takes oral chelation therapy routinely, suggests Dr. Donsbach. "The relief from these changes is within the first ten days after which no further problems should occur," he says.

The Donsbach Orachel™ formula is available from D & B Enterprises, 19400 Beach Boulevard, Suite 21, P. O. Box 5550, Huntington Beach, California 92647; telephone (714) 432-7860. The formulation is made up into small packets containing five tablets each. There are sixty packets with 300 tablets packed in a box. It is suggested that one packet be taken with breakfast and one packet be taken with dinner.

Each two packets of ten tablets contain the following ingredients and dosages:

Vitamin A (fish liver oil)	39,500 IU
Vitamin D (fish liver oil)	666 IU
Vitamin E (D-alpha tocopherol)	650 IU
Vitamin C	4,250 mg
Vitamin B-1	200 mg
Vitamin B-2	18 mg
Vitamin B-6	168 mg
Vitamin B-12	165 mcg
Niacin	80 mg
Niacinamide	18 mg
Pantothenic acid	350 mg
Folic acid	400 mcg
Biotin	100 mcg
Choline	725 mg
Inositol	40 mg
PABA	380 mg
Calcium	250 mg
Magnesium	250 mg
Iron (ferrous fumerate)	10 mg
Iodine	125 mcg
Copper	250 mcg
Zinc	28 mg
Chromium	100 mcg
Selenium	230 mcg
Potassium (citrate)	200 mg
Manganese	5 mg
Adrenal substance	50 mg
Thymus substance	50 mg
Cysteine hydrochloride	750 mg
Methionine	187.5 mg

I had mentioned earlier that Dr. Donsbach and Keith Kenyon, M.D., had formulated the Orachel™ product together. For a time they were cohosts on a Glendale, California, radio show called

"Ask the Doctor," with their product sales paying for the program. I had appeared on that program four separate times. But then the two nutritionists had a difference of opinion and broke off their association. Now Dr. Kenyon makes and distributes his own Dr. K's Orachel™, which has nearly the exact ingredients and dosages as Dr. Donsbach's product. If you prefer to deal with a physician who manufactures an oral chelating agent, you may make direct purchases by contacting Dr. Kenyon in his Glendale medical office by telephoning (213) 782-2820.

At the beginning of this chapter, I told the dramatic health restoration story of Brunson Hollingsworth. I had concluded the case history by mentioning that the patient's chelating physician, Harvey Walker, Jr., M.D., Ph.D., had prescribed Basic Prevention™ for him as one of his health maintenance oral chelators. Basic Prevention™ and other oral chelating agents are manufactured under the supervision of Dan Black, president of Advanced Medical Nutrition Inc., located at 2247 National Avenue, P. O. Box 5012, Hayward, California 94540; telephone (415) 783-6969 or outside California toll-free (800) 437-8888. All of the products that Black offers are hypoallergenic nutritional supplements to fill both the basic and specialized nutritional needs of doctors' patients. They are complementary in function to one another.

Advanced Medical Nutrition's chelating food supplements are sold for dispensing by physicians, but they are available directly to individuals in one other way. They may be purchased from the company at the established retail price when you have an authorization form signed by your health practitioner. Such a form is supplied by the company, and mailed to you when you request it. Then, you get the form approved by the doctor and can send it with your purchase order to the company's marketing manager, Janet L. Ralston, who keeps your request and its approval on file for your future nutrient needs.

Basic Prevention™ is an all-around, high-potency, multiple food supplement providing a carefully balanced foundation of vitamins, minerals, and trace elements. It features low amounts of vitamin D and no phosphorus (we get too much of both in our diet), bio-available minerals, an optimum calcium-to-magnesium ratio, and active preformed vitamin A, complemented by a full 9,000 micrograms (15,000 IU) of beta-carotene. Basic Prevention™ is available with or without copper; the doctor decides which one you need. It also can be furnished with or without raw glandular extracts for beef-sensitive or vegetarian patients.

Six tablets of Basic Prevention™ contain the following ingredients and dosages:

Vitamin A (fish liver oil)	10,000 IU
Beta-carotene	15,000 IU
Vitamin D (fish liver oil)	100 IU
Vitamin E (D-alpha-tocopherol succinate)	400 IU
Vitamin C (corn-free ascorbic acid)	1,200 IU
Vitamin B-1	100 mg
Vitamin B-2	50 mg
Vitamin B-6	100 mg
Vitamin B-12	100 mcg
Niacin	50 mg
Niacinamide	150 mg
Pantothenic acid	500 mg
Folic acid	800 mcg
Biotin	300 mcg
Choline	100 mg
Inositol	100 mg
PABA (para-amino-benzoic acid)	50 mg
Calcium (oyster shell)	500 mg
Magnesium (aspartate complex)	500 mg
Potassium (aspartate)	99 mg
Iodine (kelp)	244 mcg
Manganese (aspartate complex)	20 mg
Zinc (gluconate)	20 mg
Molybdenum (chelate, kelp)	100 mcg
Chromium (SeaSEL-1000™ kelp)	200 mcg
Selenium (SeaSEL-1000™ kelp)	200 mcg
Aspartic acid	816 mg
Bioflavonoids (rutin, hesperidin)	100 mg
SeaSEL-1000™ kelp	200 mg
Raw gland tissue (thymus/spleen/liver/adrenal = 2/2/2/1)	180 mg

The other associated oral chelators manufactured and distributed by Advanced Medical Nutrition Inc. may briefly be described in the following manner:

Redox +™ is a nutritional antioxidant formula containing the unique MSM (maxsoma saturation matrix or methylsulfonylmethane) delivery system. It additionally supplies 1-cysteine, 1-glutathione, ascorbyl palmitate, vitamin C, beta-carotene, vitamin E, and selenium.

Detoxi-Plex™ is a dietary food supplement offering extra nutritional support to help protect against environmental heavy metals and other toxins. It combines the metal-chelating activities of methionine and vitamin C with adsorptive properties of plant fibers. Yucca and sarsaparilla herbs and liver extract with high glutathione content enhance the formula.

Fiber-Plex™ capsules provide dietary fiber. Pure glucomannan fiber is combined with raw carrot powder, celery powder, high and low methoxyl pectins, alginate, and slippery elm powder. Fiber-Plex™ also comes in bulk powder.

MG-K Aspartate™, which is magnesium-potassium aspartate complex, is also available.

Aler-Gest™ is a chewable digestive enzyme that is peppermint flavored.

Neutral-C™ is pure ascorbic acid crystals buffered to a neutral pH of 7.

CHAPTER TWELVE

Pharmaceuticals, Foods, and Herbs Used for Oral Chelation Therapy

A diplomat of India visiting American relatives in New York City in early 1982, his excellency Rassi Dass of Bombay, age 62, suddenly found himself experiencing sporadic chest pains. He didn't think they were symptoms of heart disease since all his life he had eaten only healthy foods similar to the Zen macrobiotic diet. Still, he acknowledged that for the past fifteen years he had taken very little exercise, although he had been physically active as a young man. Mr. Dass also had been a student of yoga for a number of years, but not lately.

The chest pains became frequent enough that Rassi Dass was forced to seek medical attention. His relatives referred him to the World Health Medical Group in New York City where a holistic physician, Warren M. Levin, M.D., offers medical preventives with chelation therapy, nutrition, metabology, orthomolecular medicine, clinical ecology, bariatrics, and comprehensive stress management for executives. The Indian national was started on medical therapy for angina pectoris, uncontrolled hypertension, and general circulatory problems. His medical records indicate that the following drug regimen was prescribed: Inderal™, nitroglycerine, Aldomet™, diuretics, and tranquilizers.

The patient's health history states: "He has one brother who died at the age of 38 from a myocardial infarction, and he has another brother living who also has coronary artery disease. The patient experiences diminished energy and mild depression. He learned about the various therapies for coronary arteriosclerosis, but remained adamantly opposed to bypass surgery. His blood pressure is elevated at 180/130, and laboratory tests indicated an increase in his catecholamines. Additional problems include cold hands and feet, and he suffers from extreme cold sensitivity. He does not smoke nor drink alcoholic beverages."

Rassi Dass underwent a series of thirty intravenous chelation treatments, because a preliminary radionuclear stress test proved abnormal. It showed a 3 percent heart ejection fraction (the amount of blood pushed out with each heart beat) and a decreased left ventricular wall motion. Electrocardiograms also showed marked ischemic changes (local anemia due to mechanical obstruction of the heart blood supply from coronary artery narrowing) in the heart muscle near the diaphragm.

Dr. Levin, who became the patient's personal physician, kept him on the beta blocker drug, Tenormin™, for his hypertension. After being treated with twenty IV infusions of EDTA, Mr. Dass said, "I feel great." In addition, he advised the doctor, "All sorts of things about my body are better. I sleep well; I have more energy; my vision has improved; I can remember little items that once I habitually forgot." The patient continued to show steady improvement.

By the end of his series of IV infusions, the patient showed such remarkable progress in his health that Dr. Levin discharged him after putting him on a monthly maintenance program of oral chelating agents. The man remained in the United States for a few more months, but when he returned to India in December 1982, Rassi Dass carried with him an inventory of oral chelators and the addresses of future direct mail purchasing sources in the United States and around the world. As a part of his luggage, he packed sufficient supplies for years of ongoing supplementation with the following nutrients. Each day the man takes Basic Prevention™ six times, vitamin C tablets at least 3 grams, vitamin E capsules 1,600 IU, Kyolic™ (deodorized garlic) six capsules, octacosonol 3 grams, carnitine three tablets, mucopolysaccharides 3 grams, bromelain six tablets, Aspartine™ (magnesium aspartate 32 mg and potassium aspartate 90 mg) three tablets, magnesium orotate and calcium orotate each 1,500 mg, Max EPA™ (fish oil 1,000 mg) nine daily for one month and then six daily, Efamol™ (oil of evening primrose 500 mg) six capsules, six tablets of a digestive enzyme, three tablets of Liva-trophic Concentrate™, Multitrophic Chelate™ (multiple minerals) six tablets, pantothenic acid 250 mg, niacin 400 mg, N,N-dimethyl-glycine 150 mg, cod liver oil one tablespoonful twice weekly, leci-thin (about 30 grams) one tablespoonful, and Fyblend™ (high fiber powder supplement) one tablespoonful.

On his own, Rassi Dass sent away to Tokyo, Japan, for the oral chelating pharmaceutical known as Anginin™, sold over the count-er in that country as an anti-atherosclerotic agent. He made his purchase by mail order and takes the drug daily along with his nutritional chelators. All of these oral chelating agents are cardio-vascular system enhancers for the man, which he uses as surrogates for intravenous chelation therapy until he is able to locate a physi-cian near Bombay who offers intravenous injections with EDTA for invasive chelation therapy.

ORAL CHELATING DRUGS UNAPPROVED BY THE FDA

A number of pharmaceutical products manufactured overseas are available, but they are not approved by the United States Food and Drug Administration (FDA) for commercial importation into this country. Perhaps even importation for personal use into the United States is open to legal question. At least the FDA has attempted to enforce its powers against constitutional guarantees to private citi-zens who would utilize foreign drugs for their own purposes. Nev-ertheless, any American has a constitutional right to purchase and personally use medications of his own choosing. But be warned that the act of importation and distribution of an unapproved drug is liable to be a violation of the law, and such drugs are subject to seizure by the U.S. Customs authorities.

Your limitation for using non-approved oral chelators, therefore, is that you must not sell or dispense the medication to anyone else. Also, I do not condone your obtaining and making use of the drugs I am about to describe.

The public has cried out for information about oral chelating pharmaceuticals, and this causes me to comply with the demand. More than any other request, people have asked for information about drugs that do a job almost as effectively as IV chelation therapy. They want chelation therapy's benefits without the monetary expense, the number of treatments, the time it takes for each treatment, the inconvenience of traveling to chelating physicians who practice at a distance, and the unpleasantness of receiving an intravenous injection. Pleas have been made to me to investigate oral chelating drugs as a result of my publication of *Chelation Therapy*, wherein I mentioned that there are oral chelating pharmaceuticals. Then the entreaties increased when I included an entire chapter in *The Chelation Answer* on chelating yourself at home using common food substances. Those prior calls for sources of oral chelating drugs, foods, and herbs are acknowledged here and will be described in this chapter.

Anginin™ Pyridinolcarbamate: I have just explained that the Indian national Rassi Dass had acquired an exceedingly important drug chelator produced exclusively in Japan, the orally administered pyridinolcarbamate product, Anginin™. Unfortunately, the manufacturer is exceedingly slow about answering information requests. The only suggestion you might take is to be persistent in your search.

But, be cautioned that such importation of Anginin™ is possibly illegal and subject to seizure. I do not recommend that you try to import Anginin™; otherwise, I too, might be breaking the law. It is not my intent to do so.

Supplied as tablets in packages of 20 and 100, Anginin™ is clinically indicated for the relief of symptoms and prevention of the following conditions:

- Cerebral vascular diseases such as brain hemorrhage, stroke, cerebral thrombosis, senility, Alzheimer's disease, and vascular insufficiency to the brain.
- Coronary artery disease such as angina pectoris, acute myocardial infarction, and coronary insufficiency.
- Peripheral vascular diseases such as arteriosclerosis obliterans and atherosclerosis obliterans.
- Cardiac arrhythmias such as ventricular premature contraction, ventricular tachycardia, atrial fibrillation, atrial flutter, and supraventricular tachycardia.
- Angiitis (inflammation of a blood vessel) such as thromboangiitis obliterans (Buerger's disease) and Takayasu's disease.
- Purpuric states such as vascular purpura and thrombocytopenia.

- Inflammatory conditions such as osteoarthritis, rheumatic fever, and rheumatoid arthritis.
- Ophthalmic diseases such as arteriosclerotic retinopathy, diabetic retinopathy, retinal and vitreous hemorrhage, retinal vein thrombosis, uveitis, central chorioretinitis, and Behcet's disease.
- Sexual incapacities relating to interruption of the blood circulation.

For treatment of these serious diseases, the dosage range of Anginin™ is one tablet three times a day, or two tablets two or three times a day, depending upon the extent of blood vessel involvement that is diagnosed by a physician. In the treatment of hardening of the arteries and the condition's associated atherosclerotic disorders, the product brochure says that long-term self-administration should continue for at least four months with a daily dose of 0.75 to 1.5 grams (three to six tablets). As a measure to prevent hardening of the arteries, the manufacturer, Banyu Pharmaceutical Company Ltd., recommends a prophylactic dosage of one or two Anginin™ tablets a day.

Taking Anginin™ tablets regularly can result in a few side effects, but Banyu company scientists report that none of them are of a severe or serious nature. Gastric distress and loss of appetite have been experienced by a few people. In rare cases, this oral chelating drug exhibits a sensitizing reaction, such as the appearance of redness or a rash on the skin or an increase of transaminase activity in liver-function tests. In such cases of hypersensitivity, the product may be discontinued. The drug should not be utilized unless a chelating or holistic physician is first consulted about it.

With the assistance of Professor Masayuki Ishikawa, Anginin™ was synthesized in 1962 by Professor Takio Shimamoto, an important Japanese authority in the study of hardening of the arteries. The drug is a pyridine derivative, which causes it to act as a chelating agent. The product is neither a hypocholesterolemic (lowering blood cholesterol) agent or a vasodilator, although both therapeutic reactions do occur. It also pulls out noxious liquid and fatty substances from atherosclerotic plaque and helps replace atheromatous masses of material escaping from the unclogging arteries with regenerated smooth muscle cells. Anginin™ is not yet legally distributed in the United States because of current requirements for it to obtain FDA approval.

If you are interested in acquiring a supply of Anginin™ tablets for your personal use, accompanied by an eighty-page booklet describing the product, and twelve pages of medical references describing where to find medical journal articles about this drug (although you may be violating U.S. Customs law, which I say you must not do), write to Banyu Pharmaceutical Company Ltd., 7,2-chrome, Nihonbashi Honcho, Chuo-ku, Tokyo, Japan. Cable address: BANYUCO TOKYO; TELEX address: J24705 BANYUCO. Remember, I warned that your attempt may be frustrated by a long silence from the supplier. But some business news may bring improved cooperation by the Anginin™ manufacturer.

It was announced in Tokyo, on October 12, 1983, that the major American pharmaceutical manufacturer, Merck & Company, had spent $314 million to buy a controlling interest in Banyu Pharmaceutical Company. With yearly sales of more than $400 million, Banyu is among Japan's top twenty pharmaceutical marketeers. By acquiring a 50.5 percent interest in Banyu, Merck may be motivated to bring Anginin™ into the American market. It has the required $30 million in resources to meet FDA demands for laboratory research, animal research, double-blind controlled studies on humans, and other aspects of introducing a new/old drug product to the United States.

Merck's investment in Banyu is a landmark. It is the first case in history of a foreign company purchasing control of a Japanese corporation listed in the first section of the Tokyo Stock Exchange, an honor roll of that nation's established concerns. By tradition and by government policy, acquisitions are rare in Japan, and especially so when the buyer is from abroad. Perhaps Merck & Company will be more forthcoming about responding to your inquiries for Anginin™ tablets.

Lisater™: Anginin™ is also readily available in Mexico with no prescription required. It is sold in almost any drug store under the trade name Lisater™. The product is marketed under licensure of the Japanese.

Syntrival™: In the European markets, Anginin™ is available to the public, too, but under a somewhat modified formulation. It is sold as an orotate salt in combination with a highly effective and very safe nutrient known as chondroitin sulfate. The combination of Anginin™ with chondroitin sulfate is marketed in West Germany as Syntrival™. The manufacturer is Dr. Worwag Pharmazeutische Präparate, Gmb H., 7000 Strasse 55, Stuttgart 40, Unterlander, West Germany; telephone (07-11) 871012. At the November 1988 rate of 2.60 Deutch Marks (DM) to the U.S. dollar, Syntrival's™ cost is approximately DM 57.20 or $22 for 100 tablets.

The usual dosage of Syntrival™ suggested by the manufacturer is three tablets per day for three to four months and repeated later as needed.

My advice is to take no medication of this type without the consent of your medical doctor who is knowledgeable about chelation therapy and oral chelating agents.

At the same time that a person may be taking intravenous EDTA injections, the oral Anginin™ chelators such as Syntrival™ and Lisater™ could be ingested, say chelating physicians whom I have interviewed. Such oral chelating pharmaceuticals are being given by physicians around the world (except in the United States) with the reasonable expectation that benefits would be realized more rapidly during IV chelation therapy. Accordingly, the number of intravenous chelation treatments required by the patient with cardiovascular problems is decreased.

Syntrival™ is approved by the West German FDA for the reversal and treatment of arteriosclerosis including diseases of the cerebral, coronary, and peripheral body regions. Not only can an individual purchase the oral Anginin™ chelators and their combinations in West Germany, one may also acquire the injectable forms from foreign countries. Holland, for instance, is an excellent source of pharmaceutical oral chelating agents. You can buy them from almost any Dutch pharmacy with no prescription required. The manufacturer is Niederland-Enzypharm B.B. Biochemisch-Pharmaceutisch Laboratorium, 2650 Soestdijk, Dordyrtrnherhr 2-4 Post Bus 54, Niederland, Holland; telephone 0-21-55-1-24-47.

Vaso Elastin™: Niederland-Enzypharm also manufactures and sells the product Vaso Elastin™ as a highly effective injectable against hardening of the arteries. It costs $1.00 per ampule and would be quite compatible as adjunctive treatment with the invasive form of chelation therapy, or just taken by itself.

Unithiol™: Some additional new oral chelating drugs are being developed in uninterrupted worldwide research. Although most of these chelators have initially been produced for the treatment of heavy metal poisoning such as lead, mercury, and cadmium toxicity, some pharmaceuticals are finding use in the reversal of vascular disease. One of these oral chelators came out of Leningrad, U.S.S.R., and is known in Russia as Unithiol™.

Please note that I do not suggest anyone employ the product unless it has been obtained legally and your doctor approves the formulation.

The Unithiol™ formula is 2,3 dimercapto propane-1-sulfonate (DMPS). It has already been applied as oral chelation care by Russian medical investigators in conjunction with a vitamin product and was found to be therapeutic in coronary, cerebral, and peripheral vascular disease. This was reported (in *Vrach. Delo.* 6:8, 1973) by Dr. V. N. Kurliandihikov, in the article "Treatment of Patients With Coronary Arteriosclerosis With Unithiol in Combination With Decamevit." Decamevit is a multivitamin.

Unithiol™ is distributed through HEYL Chemisch-Pharmazeutische Fabrik GmbH and Company, Goerzallee 253, d-1000 Berlin 37, West Germany. It is sold as an oral chelating capsule as well as in an injectable form.

DMS: Another exciting orally effective chelating agent for the treatment of lead poisoning is currently being researched in the United States. There is a strong probability that it, too, will be found useful in the treatment of many chronic degenerative diseases, including sexual dysfunctions from arteriosclerosis. It is much safer than many of the older chelating agents that it will replace. This substance, 2,3 dimercapto succinic acid, commonly known as DMS, works effectively by mouth. It is expected to become the standard treatment in America for lead poisoning, as soon as the FDA gets around to approving it. DMS, along with the enlisting of hair analysis for early diagnosis, could usher in a new age of effective dealing with low level lead and other toxic metal excesses. For more information about DMS, contact Garry F. Gordon, M.D., medical director of his own clinic. The address and telephone number are provided in the appendix.

NTA: Research was conducted on an oral chelator known as Nitrilo Tri Acetic Acid (NTA). Martin Rubin, Ph.D., retired from

Georgetown Medical School in Washington, D.C., has shown that
NTA dissolves bladder stones in animals. When the product is completely evaluated, it may find application in several other conditions
such as hardening of the arteries.

Hexopal Forte™: Europeans are currently being treated by their
physicians with a vitamin substance that is a combination of bioflavonoids and a niacin derivative called inositol nicotinate 750 mg. I
divorce myself from suggesting that you should take inositol nicotinate without your doctor's permission. Inositol nicotinate is sold
under the name Hexopal Forte™ by Winthrop Laboratories, Ster-
ling-Winthrop House, Surbiton-Upon-Thames, Surrey, KT64PH,
England. It is used for the relief of peripheral vascular arteriosclerosis, vasospastic conditions, Raynaud's phenomenon, night cramps,
and intermittent claudication.

Paroven™: Another bioflavonoid compound is now approved for
sale in England for virtually the same indications listed for Hexopal
Forte™. Also, this new oral chelator focuses on capillary impairment
and venous insufficiency, which may be the reason for painful,
heavy, and tired legs, night cramps, varicose veins and other loose
vein states, phlebitic syndrome, hemorrhoids, and the inability to
function sexually. It repairs capillary fragility.

The product is sold under the brand name Paroven™ by Zyma
Ltd., Hurdsfield Industrial Estate, Mocclesfield, Cheshire, SK102LY,
United Kingdom. Its dosage is 250 milligrams or two to four cap-
sules taken daily for three months.

Both Paroven™ and Hexopal Forte™ are made from nutrients.
Nevertheless, they are approved in Great Britain to provide a drug-
like action in the treatment of vascular disease in the English population. Chelation-like activity is the mechanism by which they work
for therapeutic benefits.

Once again, let me emphasize that Paroven™, or any of the other
oral chelating drugs that I have informed you about, should not be
purchased and imported into the United States in violation of U.S.
Customs law. Also, you should try where possible to avoid infring-
ing on the rules and regulations of the U.S. Food and Drug Administration. The information supplied here is purely for purposes of
educating you and not an admonition that such products should or
could be applied for medical purposes by any person while he or
she is under the jurisdiction of American laws. Furthermore, such

pharmaceutical products unapproved by the FDA should never be self-administered without the supervision of a physician educated in the pharmacology and/or therapeutics of chelating drugs, since he or she has the sole authority to do such prescribing.

FOOD SUBSTANCES THAT CHELATE THE BODY

For human beings, health is a state of wholeness based on the body's ability to maintain an equilibrium between internal and external forces. Healing is the body's innate ability to restore this equilibrium and wholeness. Certain food substances, sometimes taken as food supplements, tend to maintain the body's balance so as to assure health and a continuous healing against the stressors one meets daily. Typical stressors are environmental conditions such as smog and radiation, body abuses such as smoking, eating overly processed food, and drinking alcohol, colas, and coffee, as well as the normal aging process. These stressors lead to biochemical reactions in one's body that shorten the lives of cells and thus the individual human being.

The healing food substances described in Chapters Ten and Eleven and to be described in the balance of this chapter are recognized as oral chelating agents that prolong cell life by reversing, stopping, or preventing destructive chemical reactions. They perform their minor miracles through a process of chelation therapy within the membranes of organelles. Organelles are the specialized parts of the tissue cell serving for the performance of some individual functions; these subcellular units include all types of mitochondria, the Golgi apparatus, cell center and centrioles, granular and agranular cytoplasmic reticulum, lysosomes, plasma membrane, and fibrils.

To better relate food substances to restoration of cellular destruction, refer to Figure 12.1 for a graphic illustration while I describe the anatomical physiology of cell structure. A particular source of information assisted me with the scientific aspects of what you are about to read. The nutritional supplement manufacturer, Anabolic Laboratories Inc., 17802 Gillette Avenue, Irvine, California 92714; telephone (714) 863-0340, provided scientific expertise through its technical information data sheet, "Maintenance of Cellular Integrity Through the Use of Protective Nutrients."

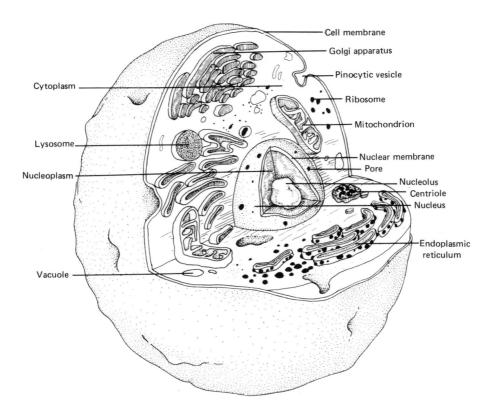

Cell membrane
Golgi apparatus
Pinocytic vesicle
Cytoplasm
Ribosome
Mitochondrion
Lysosome
Nuclear membrane
Pore
Nucleoplasm
Nucleolus
Centriole
Nucleus
Endoplasmic reticulum
Vacuole

Figure 12.1.   A Typical Animal Cell.

The human cell is comprised of hundreds of tiny chemical factories called organelles. Depicted here are many different types of organelles, each having its own
function. For example, the Golgi apparatus produces the organelles known as lysosomes.

Lysosomes are membrane-enclosed bodies that act as storage vesicles for digestive enzymes and behave like the waste-disposal mechanisms of the cell. Lysosomes have surrounding single membranes. The lysosomal membrane is imperme-
able to the outward movement of its enzymes, and is resistant to the enzymes'
digestive action. If the lysosomal membrane is ruptured by pathological organisms
or for some other reason, the enzymes released begin to immediately digest the
surrounding cytoplasm and this may destroy the cell.

Other vital organelles are the mitochondria, which serve as the cell's power-
house. The mitochondria contain two types of membranes, an outer smooth membrane and an inner membrane containing folds. The inner membrane gives rise to a
variety of enzymes that counteract the various pollutants and other stressors that
all of us meet in daily life.

The cell is the basic unit of life, the human body being made of about 80 trillion cells. (See Figure 12.1.) Each cell consists of its cytoplasm and a nucleus where DNA is located. Together they are enclosed by a sac-like membrane. The cell has many small structures within its cytoplasm called organelles. One group of the organelles is the energy-producing factories of the cell called the mitochondria. Other organelles are little sacs containing special digestive enzymes (the garbage disposal system) known as lysosomes. Then there is the endoplasmic reticulum where protein synthesis and other important processes take place.

All of these organelle structures, like the nucleus and the cell itself, are enclosed by membranes composed of lipids (fats) and proteins. (See Figure 12.2.) Altogether, they are necessary for the proper functioning of the individual cell. The membranes hold the cell and its parts together, and regulate what molecules can and cannot enter and leave the cell, the nucleus, or the organelle. In addition, organelle membranes contain very important enzymes, and receptor molecules involved in immune reaction, cell communication, and other crucial processes.

When you look carefully at Figure 12.2, you see that membranes are made of protein and saturated and unsaturated lipids which are arranged in a very intricate structure, whereby the lipids form a double layer of fat molecules. The protein molecules consisting of enzymes and receptors are dispersed throughout the double fat layer. Polyunsaturated fats are very susceptible to the formation of two types of pathology: lipid peroxidations and free radical reactions.

The destructive qualities of lipid peroxidation and free radical reaction damage membranes, thereby disrupting the normal functions that the membranes must perform in order for the cell to maintain itself. Surprisingly it is oxygen, so vital to life, that under certain conditions oxidizes unsaturated lipids to form lipid peroxides. This in itself disrupts the delicate structure of membranes, but then the peroxides break down to form free radicals, which can lead to the destruction of nearby protein molecules. To further complicate the problem, free radicals themselves initiate lipid peroxidation resulting in a vicious chain reaction. Smog, smoking, radiation, and other body abuses also produce free radicals. They tend to destroy the organelle membranes.

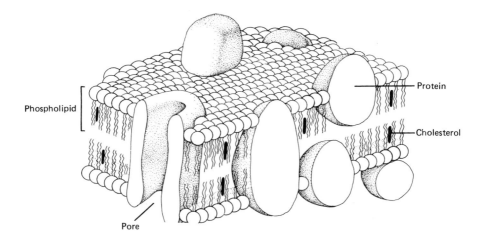

Phospholipid

Protein

Cholesterol

Pore

Figure 12.2. The Fluid-Mosaic Model of the Cell Membrane.

Correct functioning of the organelle membrane is highly significant for the health of a body cell. Alteration of the organelle membrane can seriously affect the enzyme actions within the organelle with which it is associated. It contains ion pumps, antigens, neurohumeral receptors, intercellular junctions, immunoglobulins, and other items. Damage to this intracellular (organelle) membrane can ultimately result in a biochemical disaster and end in a catastrophe of cellular illness. With membrane damage, homeostasis is lost and disease results.

Depicted here is the intracellular membrane of an organelle consisting of two layers. The top portion of phospholipids and the lower layer of cholesterol are distributed in a mosaic pattern (as a distribution of small pieces) on the surfaces and in the interior of the membrane. The lipids and proteins move laterally (to one side), so that a particular molecule found in one position during one moment may be in a different position some time later. This is a dynamic cell membrane whose structural modifications represent an adaptation to the needs of the cell.

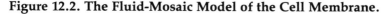

Take for example the mitochondrion organelle, which is quite susceptible to oxidative attack because of the high polyunsaturated lipid content of its membrane. If this little organelle is not maintained, the processes of electron transport, oxidative phosphorylation, and the Krebs cycle, which are all involved with the production of energy for the cell, cannot function. Then the cell will simply die.

Or consider what would happen if the cell membrane itself broke. All of the cellular components, electrolytes, and nutrients would leak out. Of recent interest is the observation that the natural aging process may involve destruction of the lysosomal membrane by free radicals, which if destroyed would cause the digestive en-zymes, usually contained within the membrane, to leak out. These enzymes would then begin to digest the cell and could diffuse out to other nearby cells and begin to destroy them, too.

Moreover, there is another process involving lysosomes. It relates to the free radical aging theory in which the presence of age pig-ments found in the heart, brain, skin, and muscles of elderly per-sons causes an inflexibility and staining of tissues. Noticed on the skin, they are often referred to as "age spots." The normal function of lysosomes is to break down either substances from the outside that the cell has taken in by phagocytosis or components of cellular waste. Lysosomes are not able to degrade peroxidized membranes properly. When they take up fragments of these chemically altered membranes, lysosomes become congested, which results in the ap-pearance of age pigments. If the lysosomes become congested, they can no longer function properly, resulting in poor functioning and eventual death of the entire cell. When enough cells have died, disease develops.

The grim story I have just laid before you might make you won-der how membranes of organelles and cells survive at all when you consider the kinds and number of polluting stressors we come in contact with daily. Fortunately nature has provided the body with natural protective systems. These include the natural body process of self-chelation, the oral chelating agents that catalyze one's own chelation mechanism, the antioxidants (substances that stop lipid peroxidation), and free radical scavengers (molecules that capture free radicals and render them harmless). All of these natural reme-dies work together to keep cells healthy. It is conceivable that taking increased amounts of cell protectors in the form of food supple-ments may not only defend the body against deleterious environ-mental conditions, but may even slow down your personal aging process.

What the chelating food substances do specifically is to protect the organelle membranes against damage from free radical pathol-ogy. Please visualize the reactions within a cellular organelle as illustrated in Figure 12.2. In *The Scientific Basis of EDTA Chelation Therapy*, Dr. Halstead explains: "The organelle's membrane proteins may interact with membrane lipids to launch biochemical reactions, evoking a series of messengers to other membrane-bound structures within a cell. This results in a physiologic response. The general topography of membranes includes well-defined structural and functional sites, including ion pumps, antigens, neurohumerol receptors, intercellular junctions, immunoglobulins, and other structures. This is why damage to intracellular membranes can ultimately result in a biochemical disaster and terminate in a health catastrophe."

With exposure to carcinogens, pathogens, pollutants, mutagens, allergens, atherogens, poisonous heavy metals, and other assaults on our bodies that people meet every day, as I pointed out previously, free radicals are created in the tissues. Dr. Halstead repeats, "Free radicals can adversely affect cellular health by producing lipid peroxidation of intracellular membranes [as shown in Figure 12.2]. Organelles such as mitochondria and lysosomes, which control cellular metabolism, are membrane-enclosed bags of enzymes. When these membranes are damaged, cellular homeostasis is altered, and disease results."

But the chelating food substances, oral chelating pharmaceuticals, intravenously administered chelating drugs such as EDTA, chelating herbs, chelating enzymes, and other agents assist in inhibiting lipid peroxidation by removing metal ions, such as calcium, iron, and copper, which are present in the process of lipid peroxidation. In this way, chelating substances that you may take into your body help to maintain cellular homeostasis and the state of health and wholeness that all of us find desirable.

When I spoke of Syntrival™ in the previous section on oral chelating pharmaceuticals, I mentioned that this drug is unique by its chondroitin sulfate content. Chondroitin sulfate is a mucopolysaccharide, a natural dietary ingredient. Knowledgeable and interested physicians who use nutrition as therapy are currently acting to get mucopolysaccharides approved by the FDA. A nutrition-pharmaceutical company has been incorporated in the United States for accomplishing this approval as treatment against hardening of the arteries.

Mucopolysaccharides: Comprising part of the structure of cartilage tissue such as in the ear or nose of an animal or in the New Zealand green-lipped mussel or in some plants, mucopolysaccharides may be swallowed as tableted food supplements readily obtained from health food stores. A textbook published by Charles

C. Thomas of Springfield, Illinois, *Coronary Heart Disease and the Mucopolysaccharides (Glycosaminoglycans),* by Lester Morrison, M.D., discusses the exciting research going on in this field. Dr. Morrison was director and research professor at the Institute for Arteriosclerosis Research, Loma Linda University School of Medicine. He has become the guru of mucopolysaccharides in medicine.

In another book published by St. Martin's Press of New York City, *Dr. Morrison's Heart-Saver Program,* the elderly medical researcher provides an anti-atherosclerotic food formula consisting of ten ingredients: soya lecithin, phosphatidylcholine, phosphatidyl inositol, phosphatidyl ethanolamine, LipoStabil™ or "Lethicon" (a special form of lecithin), extract of Irish moss, extract of carrageenan, silicon dioxide, niacin, and mucopolysaccharides. Mucopolysaccharides (MPS) is the main nutritive set of ingredients in the Morrison formula bringing about a therapeutic effect for counteracting heart and blood vessel diseases.

MPS "are primarily carbohydrates linked to protein," states Dr. Morrison. "I say 'primarily' because there are many MPS from many sources, and they have many variations in structure."

Mucopolysaccharides are also known as glycosaminoglycans, which are complexes of protein and polysaccharides in which the polysaccharide component is generally a major part of the complex. MPS comprise much of the ground substances of connective tissue in animals and plants. When there is a disruption in MPS metabolism, the resulting diseases include various defects of bone, cartilage, and connective tissue.

Writing in the clinical journal, *Applied Nutrition in Clinical Practice,* in 1973, Orville Miller, Ph.D., of the School of Pharmacy, University of Southern California, defined MPS this way:

> Mucopolysaccharides play a major role in the structural integrity of all body tissues and are largely responsible for the form and organization of the human system as components of connective tissue. They have aptly been described as the "glue of life." They are involved in transfer of electrolytes and nutrients through cell walls. Mucopolysaccharides occur in the organic matrix of bone and teeth and function in both a structural and nutritional capacity. They are also largely responsible for the elasticity of skin and of blood vessels.

Soybean Lecithin: Lecithin comprises about 30 percent of brain matter and is concentrated in tissues of the liver, heart, spleen, ovaries, testicles, and thyroid. It acts as a powerful emulsifier of fats and oils in the body including cholesterol, and has a key role in preventing fatty deposits in blood vessels, which are factors in heart disease.

Lecithin in daily foods such as that derived from soybeans (the healthiest kind) is broken down into its various constituents during digestion in the same way proteins are reduced into the different amino acids. Choline and inositol are liberated in this process. Enzymes engineer the task of rebuilding sufficient lecithin within body cells. Our bodies can make enough lecithin for daily use as an emulsifier of blood stream fats.

Since our bodies make their own lecithin, the FDA prohibits the inclusion of lecithin in multiple vitamin-mineral products as a food supplement. But cooking oils and overprocessing of foods destroy certain lecithin-making nutrients. For instance, choline, inositol, magnesium, pyridoxine, and methionine must be present in suitable amounts for the body to create its own lecithin. It makes good sense, therefore, to supplement, preferably with soya lecithin, to provide all of the primary ingredients for a healthy body.

MaxEPA™ Omega-3 Fatty Acids: For decades researchers have been trying to reconcile the role of cholesterol and fats in heart disease. Even though animal fats contain some polyunsaturated fats and vegetables contain some saturated fats, vegetable oils have been recommended by the American Heart Association for consumption by the public rather than animal fats. An enigmatic situation has prevailed, however, with Eskimos who consume a diet rich in animal fat yet are virtually free of heart disease. Japanese fishermen also suffer fewer coronaries than Westerners. The one common factor to both the Eskimos and Japanese is that they subsist largely on a diet of cold-water fatty fish. When herring, haddock, cod, and mackerel are abundantly added to Western diets, blood changes occur in consumers that mimic the protective blood of the Eskimo and the Japanese fisherman.

Since most North Americans and Europeans easily tire of daily rations of fatty fish, extracts were prepared to see if the same beneficial results could be achieved. The specially selected marine lipids concentrated in a product called MaxEPA™ did produce the beneficial results. MaxEPA™ protects against heart disease and strokes; benefits the function of glands and enzymes; improves brain and nerve structures; and treats systemic lupus erythematosus, arthritis and other autoimmune syndromes, and certain conditions of the kidneys. Its action is due primarily to two nutrients, both of which are a class of long-chained, polyunsaturated fatty acids called "omega-3." One of the nutrients is eicosapentaenoic acid (EPA), which is required for the production of prostaglandin-3, a hormone-like substance that controls blood clotting and arterial spasms. EPA also improves blood viscosity, lowers cholesterol blood levels, and reduces serum triglycerides. The other nutrient, docosahexaenoic acid (DHA), is a major component of the brain and retinal tissue and has a possible role in nerve transmission.

Each MaxEPA™ gelatin capsule is 1,000 milligrams (1 gram) and contains 18 percent EPA, 12 percent DHA, 0.1 percent free fatty acids, 100 IU per gram of vitamin A, and 1 IU per gram of vitamin E. The usual bottle quantity is 100 capsules.

MaxEPA™ omega-3 fatty acids may be purchased as a food supplement from a health food store, or go right to the manufacturer's sales manager, Robert Fredericks, the R. P. Scherer Company of North America Inc., 2725 Sherer Drive, St. Petersburg, Florida 33702; telephone (813) 576-4000.

N,N-Dimethylglycine: Neither a vitamin nor a food additive, N,N-dimethylglycine (DMG) has been designated a non-fuel nutrient. In contrast with "fuel" nutrients that supply energy to the body for all its needs through the breakdown of carbohydrates, fats, and proteins, a "non-fuel" nutrient, such as a vitamin or mineral, is required by the body in small amounts for catalyzing internal chemical reactions but not for energy use. DMG works inside the human body as part of the biochemical pathway, which is where chemical substances support living tissue. As part of this pathway, DMG is manufactured by the body, and it is also found as a natural, non-toxic component of some foods, such as cereal grains, sugar beets, sunflower seeds, organ meats, and apricot pits. Nutritional researchers have reported that supplementation with DMG increases cellular efficiency and helps to combat fatigue, lack of oxygen in the tissues, alcoholism, diabetes mellitus, atherosclerosis, sexual dysfunction, and more.

DMG accomplishes its benefits by being a "methyl donor." A methyl group is a molecular fragment consisting of one carbon and three hydrogen atoms, which are bonded together. DMG gives up these methyl groups through a process called oxidative demethylation via indirect transmethylation. In this biochemical process, one-carbon units, such as the methyl group, are transferred from one molecule to another. By making this methyl donation, DMG aids vitamins, fats, hormones, and proteins in completing their metabolic action. It is through the same process (transmethylation) that DMG detoxifies the membranes present in cellular organelles.

The effects of this transmethylation lead to an increase of oxygen utilization by cellular tissue. All body cells need oxygen to function, and by assisting the oxygenation process, DMG significantly affects health problems for the better.

With this scientific background, you may understand that DMG is an "intermediary metabolite" of the choline cycle and is considered a "metabolic enhancer." It increases your state of well-being by increasing the efficiency of operations within the cell.

At present, no category exists within official government standards for what DMG is. As a result, the U.S. Food and Drug Administration has given the various DMG manufacturers a really hard time about their statements relating to the physical benefits that may be experienced from taking the product. N,N-dimethylglycine may be purchased in health food stores under the brand name Aangamik DMG™, which is a product of FoodScience Laboratories, Dominick Orlandi, President, 20 New England Drive, Essex Junction, Vermont 05452; telephone (802) 878-5508 or toll-free outside of Vermont (800) 451-5190. FoodScience furnishes DMG as tiny, white, 90-milligram pills that melt under the tongue. Each tablet is packaged in foil, attached in foiled sheets, and boxed.

Protomorphogens: Protomorphology is the scientific use of enzymes and their activators, which are protomorphogens. Protomorphogens are proteins that come from each cell. Another way to describe them is as fractional blueprints that determine what the cell is going to build before it does any building. They are the catalyzers of protein synthesis such as the germ cells (sperm and egg), along with other building blocks that make up the whole person, present as specialized components of every cell. Offspring carry the characteristics of the parents, which are delivered by means of these blueprint substances. Protomorphogens originate in each of the cells of the body and are carried by the bloodstream to the gonads for assembly. The cell's blueprint substances, protomorphogens, are non-vitamin food factors and essential components of the body's enzymatic-protein construction. In the form of enzymes and determinants, they promote the formation of a layer of protein molecules on the outer cell wall. They build and repair the cell, especially its organelles, when it comes under stress. During the continuous process of growth and repair, the cell wall is rebuilt outside this protein layer. The guidance for cell construction is accomplished by the aggregate of enzymes, trace minerals, and other nutrients furnished from what you eat.

You can eat raw organ parts of animals and take in protomorphogens. They don't have to be created by your body's own structure. An aspect of oral chelation therapy is eating simple extracts of various raw glandular tissues. They are extra protomorphogens in the form of glandular extracts of meats manufactured and distributed by nutritional laboratories as plain tablets, enteric-coated tablets, capsules, droplets, or powders for self-help. They are also dispensed by pharmacies on prescription from holistic physicians. The glandular factors involved in dietary supplementation have always been present in foods in the same way as vitamins; now they have also been concentrated as food supplements.

The glandular systems are directly involved in every function of the bodily processes. Specific nutritional support of these glands, then, becomes of utmost importance in the restoration and preservation of health. In many of the oral chelating formulas shown in Chapter Eleven, you will observe that raw glandular extracts are present in the form of thymus, adrenal, brain, heart, kidney, liver, pancreas, lung, orchic, ovarian, spleen, duodenum, or other substances. You may receive information about these extracts from their manufacturers or distributors. The makers of protomorphogen raw glandular substances are the following:

Nutri-Dyn/Micro-Dyn
Jeff Katke, President
23151 Alcalde Drive, Suite B-4
Laguna Hills, California 92653
(714) 855-1718

Nutri-Dyn Products
1907 North Britain
Dallas, Texas 75061
(214) 438-9660

Nutri-Dyn Products Corporation
5705 West Howard Street
Niles, Illinois 60648
(312) 647-0350

Standard Process Laboratories Inc.
Division of Vitamin Products Company
P. O. Box 662
2023 West Wisconsin Avenue
Milwaukee, Wisconsin 53201
(414) 933-2100

V. M. Nutri Food Inc.
P. O. Box 286
1012 Host Drive
Lake Geneva, Wisconsin 53147
(414) 248-1006

Spirulina: A small alga, which is a unique vegetable plankton that grows naturally in alkaline waters and is cultivated and harvested in hygienic tanks and ponds under scientific conditions, is made into a food supplement. It is called spirulina. This fresh water algae has the highest conversion rate of sunlight—8 percent—as compared to other plants (3 to 5 percent). Thus spirulina brings you the most potent form of nutritional benefits derived from photosynthesis of the sun's light. It is a complete vegetable protein and is the source of practically all the vitamins, minerals, digestive enzymes, trace elements, cell salts, and chlorophyll your body needs for almost perfect nutrition.

For purposes of bringing you the most complete information about the subject, I went to visit with the ultimate expert on spirulina, Christopher Hills, Ph.D., D.Sc., who is president of the Microalgae International Union and chief executive officer of Aquaculture Nutrition Products Company, P. O. Box 867, Boulder Creek, California 95006; telephone (408) 338-4827. Dr. Hills pointed out that the spirulina algae are the richest source of natural protein yet found, containing 60 to 71 percent protein, of which 37 percent (a bit less than dried egg, but more than dried skimmed milk, brewer's yeast, or soy flour) is usable. It is loaded with beta-carotene and has all eight essential amino acids, without cholesterol.

Included in spirulina's 8 percent fat content is gamma-linolenic acid, which previously has only been found in human milk and the herbal oil of evening primrose (which I will discuss next). Research indicates that gamma-linolenic acid is valuable in treating an assortment of physical problems.

Essential minerals in spirulina include iron, magnesium, manganese, zinc, potassium, and others. It has only a trace of vitamin C, which is added in the form of sodium ascorbate during processing to preserve the nutritional value of the algae. Other vitamins present in larger amounts are all of the B complex, especially B-12, so that spirulina could be an important food supplement for vegetarians. Only four tablets provide more than 6,000 IU of vitamin A. One tablespoonful has one and a half times more niacin than a half-cup serving of brown rice. The plant is so packed with power, in fact, that the authority says you could actually live on just two to three teaspoonfuls a day. It is concentrated nutrition.

Spirulina is available in tablet form, as pure spirulina, or it may be combined with other nutritional substances such as ginseng, brewer's yeast, bee pollen, papaya enzyme, niacin, calcium gluconate, pyridoxine, and other ingredients. It also is packaged in jars and tins as 100 percent spirulina powder for mixing into juices, blender drinks, sprinkling over salads, and serving in other ways. Full books of recipes have been written on how to enjoy this microalgae as part of your food supply.

The number and variety of chelating type nutrients in spirulina is immense. The chemical analysis of spirulina by the United Nations Laboratories in Table 12.1 is just a partial listing.

Dr. Hills suggests that there is no need to purchase quantities of N,N-Dimethylglycine, because he says, "Eating calcium gluconate, niacin, and spirulina all at the same time activates the cellular metabolite responsible for the biological action associated with DMG.

Table 12.1   Chemical Analysis of Spirulina

Essential Amino Acid	Percentage	Non-Essential Amino Acid	Percentage
Isoleucine	4.13%	Alanine	5.82%
Leucine	5.80%	Arginine	5.98%
Lysine	4.00%	Aspartic acid	6.43%
Methionine	2.17%	Cystine	0.67%
Phenylalanine	3.95%	Glutamic acid	8.94%
Threonine	4.17%	Glycine	3.46%
Tryptophan	1.13%	Histidine	1.08%
Valine	6.00%	Proline	2.97%
		Serine	4.00%
		Tyrosine	4.60%
Vitamin	**mg/kg**	**Mineral**	**mg/kg**
Biotin	0.4 mg/kg	Calcium	1,315 mg/kg
Vitamin B-12	2.0 mg/kg	Phosphorus	8,942 mg/kg
Pantothenic acid	11.0 mg/kg	Iron	580 mg/kg
Folic acid	0.5 mg/kg	Sodium	412 mg/kg
Inositol	350.0 mg/kg	Chloride	4,400 mg/kg
Nicotinic acid	118.0 mg/kg	Magnesium	1,915 mg/kg
Vitamin B-6	3.0 mg/kg	Manganese	25 mg/kg
Vitamin B-1	55.0 mg/kg	Zinc	39 mg/kg
Vitamin B-2	40.0 mg/kg	Potassium	15,400 mg/kg
Vitamin E	190.0 mg/kg	Others	57,000 mg/kg

So the nutrient is naturally created in our stomachs without buying any special synthetic preparation."

Aquaculture Nutrition Products Company, the Hills spirulina research organization, distributes its products through a multilevel marketing arm called the Light Force Company. If you wish to be associated with Light Force as a distributor or want to buy spirulina products for your personal consumption, you can fill your need by contacting Deborah Rozman, Aquaculture's executive vice president, or Douglas Grey, the marketing manager of the Light Force Company, at P. O. Box N, Boulder Creek, California 95006; telephone (408) 462-5000.

The holistic approach to health is steadily gaining prominence as a result of many new scientific discoveries in the areas of nutrition. Along the way, medical researchers have rediscovered the powerful benefits of herbs that have always grown around us. All plants are herbs, whether they grow on the land or in the sea. To the extent that you and I consume vegetables, fruits, spices, grains, and other vegetation, we are already using herbs as nutritional sources. There are, however, a great many herbs that contain medical properties. They have not been entirely available to the general population simply because most allopathic physicians have been ignorant of their medicinal uses. It is only recently that chelating physicians, who are more open to accepting new health care approaches, have been employing certain herbs for their oral chelating effects. Three herbs or herbal combinations fit this category of being chelators: oil of evening primrose, garlic, and Adaptrin™.

Oil of Evening Primrose: The herb oil of evening primrose is the only source—other than mother's milk—of both linoleic acid and gamma-linolenic acid (GLA), something I mentioned when discussing spirulina. These two acids help your body to manufacture the beneficial compounds I have identified in the section on MaxEPA™ as prostaglandins, which regulate a wide range of body functions including blood pressure, blood clotting, healthy skin, cholesterol levels, and hormone response.

At the October 28-30, 1983, Reno, Nevada meeting of the American College of Advancement in Medicine, I listened to David Horrobin, Ph.D., of the Institute for Innovative Medicine, Montreal, Canada, discuss evening primrose oil. There are over seventy species of the evening primrose plant that are grown for medicinal purposes from special stocks of seed reserved for production of high-grade oil. Taken as a dietary supplement of essential fatty acids, evening primrose oil has been found necessary for cell structure growth. Its essential fatty acid content compared with any other vegetable oil is higher in linoleic acid, which is converted in the body to GLA, a primary source of longer chain polyunsaturates and of the prostaglandins. If conversion in your body to GLA happens to be reduced due to illness, the deficiency can be corrected by supplementing with capsules containing oil of evening primrose. The dietary GLA is then available in the body for onward conversion by natural processes to the important longer-chain structural fatty acids and prostaglandins.

Depending on the brand of oil of evening primrose, its capsules contain 500 to 600 milligrams of nutrient, comprised of about 70-percent-by-weight linoleic acid. Quest Vitamin Supplies Ltd. can supply these nutritional capsules. Quest Vitamin Supplies distributes Naudicelle™ capsules made by Bio-Oil Research Ltd. of Crewe, England; Naudicelle™ provides 600 milligrams of evening primrose oil with a suggested dosage of six capsules to be taken daily.

An even more effective evening primrose oil product is Quest Gamma Oil Premium™ with over 10 percent natural GLA—more than any other brand on the market. The Quest product is extracted from exclusive hybrid seed stock developed over years of research. Advanced technology concerning nitrogen extraction and full pharmaceutical specifications have produced the highest quality, most potent evening primrose oil available. Quest Gamma Oil Premium™ is packaged and distributed in the United States by Montana Naturals International Inc., 19994 Highway 93, Arlee, Montana 59821; telephone (406) 726-3214. Or, you may acquire a quantity directly from Barrie Carlson, President, Quest Vitamin Supplies Ltd., 312-8495 Ontario Street, Vancouver, British Columbia V5X 3E8, Canada; telephone (604) 261-0611. You can also write to 511 King Street West, Suite 302, Toronto, Ontario M5V 1K4, Canada; telephone (416) 593-5345.

Efamol™, another English evening primrose oil product, is distributed by Nature's Way Products Inc., Ken Murdock, President, 1400 Mountain Springs Parkway, Springville, Utah 84663; telephone (800) 832-6697, (800) 962-8873, or (801) 489-3631. Efamol™ contains 500 milligrams of evening primrose oil, which supplies 40 milligrams of gamma-linolenic acid, 350 milligrams of linoleic acid, and 13 IU vitamin E.

Kyolic™: Garlic, *Allium sativum*, another chelating herb, has plenty of empirical and clinical evidence to prove its effectiveness both in prevention and treatment of disease. But raw garlic has a strong oxidizing agent in it called allicin, which gives off an unpleasant odor. A nutrition-minded firm, the Wakunaga Pharmaceutical Company of Osaka, Japan, through its American subsidiary, Wakunaga of America Inc., produces and distributes a deodorized garlic, Kyolic™, in tablets, capsules, and liquid that modifies the allicin by means of a secret aging process. The processing changes allicin from a potentially harmful oxidizer to an antioxidant so that Kyolic™ then increases energy production for mitochondria and has a binding action with lead, mercury, and cadmium. The latter property makes Kyolic™ an oral chelating agent.

There are certain therapeutically "identified factors" in raw garlic including:

- Allicin, the substance that makes garlic antibacterial and anti-inflammatory but causes the herb's unpleasant odor. Kyolic™ has eliminated the odor and made eating the herb as a food supplement socially acceptable and quite therapeutic.
- Allin, a sulfur-containing amino acid from which garlic makes allicin by the action of the enzyme allinase, gives the herb its antibiotic effect.
- Gurwitch rays, a mitogenetic radiation factor, stimulates cell growth and rejuvenates body functions.
- Anti-hemolytic factor is responsible for garlic's beneficial treatment of anemia.
- Anti-arthritic factor reduces joint inflammation and swelling.
- Sugar metabolism factor makes garlic useful for treating diabetes and hypoglycemia.
- Allithiamine is formed by the action of vitamin B-1 on allin to act as a tonic for well-being.
- Selenium is packed into garlic and provides its anti-atherosclerotic and anticancer properties by preventing platelet adhesion and blood clot formation.
- A detoxification effect neutralizes heavy metal poisons and improves the functioning of the liver, kidneys, nervous system, and circulatory system.
- Antioxidant factor allows garlic, like onions, marjoram, and green chillies, to reduce lipid peroxides and free radicals.

All of the benefits of blood purification and other properties of garlic are now available with use of the food supplement. Swallowed daily, six Kyolic™ tablets or capsules of 270 milligrams each furnish a chelating effect to the tissue cells. The Kyolic™ formula is packaged in bottles of 100 or 200 tablets, 100 or 200 capsules, two or four fluid ounces of liquid with 62 or 124 gelatin capsules, respectively, and with or without vitamin B-1. The tablets and the capsules are also blended with brewer's yeast (27 milligrams), kelp (9 milligrams), and algin (9 milligrams). The capsules alone with 220 milligrams of garlic extract powder are blended with calcium lactate (200 milligrams) and vitamin C (100 milligrams). Also there are Kyolic™ tablets with no brewer's yeast containing 9 milligrams of algin and

300 milligrams of Kyolic™. These Kyolic™ products may be acquired in most health food stores or your can get your supply by contacting the company directly. Write or telephone sales manager Charles Fox, Wakunaga of America Ltd., 23501 Madero Drive, Mission Viejo, California 92691; telephone (714) 855-2776 or toll-free inside California (800) 544-5800 or toll-free outside of California (800) 421-2998.

Adaptrin™: Clinically tested in Switzerland, a combination of twenty-two wild-picked and organically grown herbs exert a diverse range of healing effects by correcting the balance of the body's own production of prostaglandins. Adaptrin™ is an oral chelator that was once called Padma 28™. It also alters the interaction of thrombocytes and enhances the immunological and circulatory systems. Toxicity testing has established that it is completely non-toxic, has no side effects, and does not interact with other drugs.

Adaptrin™ is a Tibetin camphorin combination formula and may be used as an oral chelating preventive agent or as a remedy to reverse existing disease. The preventive and maintenance dosage is one tablet twice daily. In order to maintain its effectiveness over a long period of use, you will find it advantageous to discontinue ingestion of the herbal combination every few months for a period of one week. The recommended dosage for therapeutic chelation therapy is to take two tablets two times a day. It is advisable to start out with two tablets daily and gradually build up to the maximum dosage over the course of three weeks. The tablets should be swallowed at least one half hour before or one hour after meals. The product comes in bottles of sixty tablets (a fifteen- to thirty-day supply). Beneficial effects are often reported within two weeks.

You may acquire a quantity of Adaptrin™ by contacting George Weissman, Ph.D., President, or J. Travis Burgeson, Marketing Director, Central Health Network, 2124 Kittredge Street, Suite E, Berkeley, California 94709; telephone (415) 548-6769 or toll-free inside California (800) 262-8555 or outside California (800) 223-8555.

Honeybee Pollen: Research indicates that honeybee pollen is one of nature's most complete foods and contains virtually every known vitamin (including the entire B complex), mineral, and amino acid required for health and energy. Indeed, because most essential nutrients are found in bee pollen and are balanced by nature, it works synergistically, even in small amounts, to correct the chemical imbalance in the body after exertion. You restore yourself quicker with bee pollen as part of your food supply.

In Chapter Ten, I told the amazing story of the active Mr. Noel Johnson of San Diego, now 90, who has slowed his aging down to a crawl while he runs marathons, defends his senior boxing title, dances almost nightly, and sexually satisfies much younger women. One of his nutritional secrets, Johnson revealed, is that he eats a daily quantity of honeybee pollen supplied by Royden Brown, owner of the C. C. Pollen Company of Scottsdale, Arizona.

Bee pollen should be considered in any nutritional and energy building program. In fact, Olympic-class athletes, including Steve Riddick, a world-class U.S. sprinter, have claimed publicly that using bee pollen increases their resistance to fatigue and improves stamina. Energy begets energy, and one of the reasons honeybee pollen is thought to be such a positive source of energy is due to its rapid assimilation and use by the body. Laboratory tests show traces of bee pollen in the blood and urine only two hours after ingestion. The constant dragged-out feeling of chronic fatigue that may keep you from seriously considering exercising can be alleviated. Honeybee pollen is nature's own super-starter for unlocking your energy.

You may acquire your share of honeybee pollen packaged as High-Desert® Chewable PollenS™ (tablets), Fresh High-Desert™ Granules (flakes) in refrigerated heat-sealed poly bags, Nitrogen-Canned High-Desert® PollenS™ in table-top shaker half-pound or one-pound cans, Bee-Thin® Diet Wafers, or perhaps even bee pollen carob-coated bars. To try out these products, contact the president of C.C. Pollen Company, Bruce Brown, 6900 East Camelback Road, Suite 530, Scottsdale, Arizona 85251; telephone (602) 947-8011. C. C. Pollen also makes a bee pollen product for dogs and cats called Pet Power™.

Bromelain: An enzyme found in fresh pineapple, bromelain provides a chelation-like effect similar to using a pipe-cleaner on the blood vessels. It helps to prevent clogging of the coronary arteries that contributes to angina and heart attacks by reducing inflammation that comes with blood vessel irritation, especially phlebitis. Bromelain assists in thinning the blood, delaying red blood cells in their clumping action, and lowering the risk of blood clots. It also works in the tissue cells by selectively increasing membrane permeability so that other nutrients taken as oral chelators can get into the tissues faster. Besides pineapple, bromelain is found in many other fresh tropical fruits. If for some reason you are prevented from eating quantities of tropical fruits, you can supplement with bromelain tablets purchased from the health food store.

Papain: From the papaya, a large plant growing in tropical climates, the enzyme papain acts similar to bromelain as an oral chelating agent. It helps to break down protein by proteolytic action and improves the cellular membranes' passage of liquids.

APPENDIX
Chelating Physicians Worldwide

The physicians recorded here who offer patients intravenous (IV) chelation therapy follow the protocol of the American College of Advancement in Medicine, and many but not all of them have been certified as chelating physicians by the American Board of Chelation Therapy.

This listing is based on the membership directory of the American College of Advancement in Medicine (ACAM) and is published with ACAM's permission. A key giving information about each physician is provided before the list. For an updated directory or the most current listing of ACAM doctors in a particular geographic region, contact the American College of Advancement in Medicine, 23121 Verdugo Drive, Suite 204, Laguna Hills, California 92653; (714) 585-7666 within California or (800) 532-3688 outside California.

Members of the American College of Advancement in Medicine include diplomates (indicated by **DIPL**), diplomate candidates (indicated by **D/C**), and licensed physicians who administer chelation therapy in accordance with ACAM's protocol (indicated by **P**).

A **diplomate** of the American Board of Chelation Therapy is an individual who:

1. Is a graduate of an approved school of medicine (D.O. or M.D., or foreign equivalent);
2. Is currently licensed to practice in the state or territory where he/she conducts practice;

3. Has been recommended (by letter) by two diplomates in chelation therapy;
4. Has successfully completed the written examination of the American Board of Chelation Therapy;
5. Shows evidence of being responsible for the administration of 1,000 chelation treatments;
6. Has satisfied the requirements for preceptor training as outlined in the protocol of preceptorship;
7. Has successfully completed the oral examination of the American Board of Chelation Therapy;
8. Submits ten acceptable questions and answers with references for use in future written exams.

A **diplomate candidate** of the American Board of Chelation Therapy is an individual who:

1. Is a graduate of an approved school of medicine (D.O. or M.D. or foreign equivalent);
2. Is currently licensed to practice in the state or territory where he/she conducts practice;
3. Has been recommended (by letter) by two diplomates in chelation therapy;
4. Has successfully completed the written examination of the American Board of Chelation Therapy, and is in the process of completing the remaining requirements for ABCT diplomate status.

To get in touch with the American College of Advancement in Medicine, contact one of the following:

ACAM HEADQUARTERS ADMINISTRATIVE STAFF

Edward A. Shaw, Ph.D.
Executive Director
23121 Verdugo Drive, #204
Laguna Hills, CA 92653
(714) 583-7666 or (800) 532-3688

Sally Bonebrake
Administrative Services Coordinator

Grace Claus
Membership Services Coordinator

HEADQUARTERS ADDRESS

American College of Advancement in Medicine
23121 Verdugo Drive, Suite 204
Laguna Hills, California 92653
(714) 583-7666
(800) 532-3688 (National)

Please note that this directory of chelating physicians and/or physicians who practice holistic medicine may not be republished, reprinted, sold, or duplicated in whole or in part in any form or by any means for any commercial purpose or for the compilation of mailing lists without the prior written permission of this book's author or the American College of Advancement in Medicine.

Key to Worldwide American College of Advancement in Medicine Physician's List

PROFESSIONAL LEVEL CODES

DIP Diplomate of the American Board of Chelation Therapy
D/C Diplomate candidate of the American Board of Chelation Therapy
P   Licensed physician member of the American College of Advancement in Medicine who administers chelation therapy in accordance with the ACAM protocol.

SPECIALTY CODES

A	Allergy	IM	Internal Medicine
AN	Anesthesiology	LM	Legal Medicine
AC	Acupuncture	MM	Metabolic Medicine
AR	Arthritis	NT	Nutrition
AU	Auriculotherapy	OBS	Obstetrics
BA	Bariatrics	OME	Orthomolecular Medicine
CD	Cardiovascular	OPH	Ophthalmology
CT	Chelation Therapy	OSM	Osteopathic Manipulation
CS	Chest Disease	PD	Pediatrics
DD	Degenerative Disease	PM	Preventive Medicine
DIA	Diabetes	PMR	Physical Medicine &
END	Endocrinology		Rehabilitation
FP	Family Practice	P	Psychiatry
GE	Gastroenterology	PO	Psychiatry Orthomolecular
GP	General Practice	PH	Public Health
GER	Geriatrics	PUD	Pulmonary Diseases
GYN	Gynecology	R	Radiology
HGL	Hypoglycemia	RHU	Rheumatology
HO	Hyperbaric Oxygen	RHI	Rhinology
HOM	Homeopathy	S	Surgery
HYP	Hypnosis	WR	Weight Reduction

American College of Advancement in Medicine (ACAM) Physicians—United States

ALABAMA

Birmingham

P. Gus J. Prosch Jr., M.D. **(P)**
759 Valley St.
Birmingham, AL 35226
(205) 823-6180
A, AR, CT, GP, NT, OME

Cottonwood

H. Ray Evers, M.D. **(P)**
P. O. Drawer 587
Cottonwood, AL 36320
(205) 691-2161
(800) 621-8924 (Nat)
CT, DD, NT, MM, PM

Huntsville

George Gray, M.D. **(P)**
204 Lowe Bldg. 2, Ste 7
Huntsville, AL 35801
(205) 533-4464
IM, GER, BA, PM, NT, CT

Pat Hamm, M.D. **(P)**
3804 6th Ave.
Huntsville, AL 35807
(205) 534-8115
AR, CD, CT, DD, NT, PM, P

ALASKA

Anchorage

F. Russel Manuel, M.D. **(P)**
4120 Laurel St., Ste 106
Anchorage, AK 99508
(907) 562-6070
CT, GP, PM

Robert Rowen, M.D. **(DIPL)**
615 East 82nd Ave., Ste 300
Anchorage, AK 99518
(907) 344-7775
AC, CT, FP, PM, HYP

Soldotna

Paul G. Isaak, M.D.
Box 219
Soldotna, AK 99669
(907) 262-9341
(Retired)

Wasilla

Robert E. Martin, M.D. **(D/C)**
P. O. Box 870710
Wasilla, AK 99687
(907) 376-5284
AU, CT, FP, GP, OS, PM

ARIZONA

Lake Havasu City

Francis J. Woo Jr., M.D. **(P)**
60 Riviera Drive
Lake Havasu City, AZ 86404
(602) 453-3330
A,CT,P,GER,PM

Mesa

DeWall J. Hildreth, D.O. **(P)**
4830 East Main St., Ste 27
Mesa, AZ 85205
(602) 832-3014
CT,DD,PM

Gordon H. Josephs, D.O. **(P)**
1135 N. Mesa Dr., Ste 14
Mesa, AZ 85201
(602) 464-2086
CT,GP,GER,NT,PM

Phoenix

Stanley R. Olsztyn, M.D. **(P)**
Whitton Place
3610 N. 44th St., Ste 210
Phoenix, AZ 85018
(602) 954-0811
A,CT,PM,DD

Scottsdale

Terry S. Friedmann, M.D. **(D/C)**
7315 E. Evans Road
Scottsdale, AZ 85260
(602) 443-1409
A,CT,FP,HGL,HYP,NT

Gordon H. Josephs, D.O. **(P)**
7129 E. Mercer Lane
Scottsdale, AZ 85254
(602) 998-9234
CT,GP,NT,PM,S

ARKANSAS

Dumas

Robert A. Hoagland, M.D. **(D/C)**
145 W. Waterman
Dumas, AR 71639
(501) 382-4878
FP,OBS,S

Leslie

Melissa Taliaferro, M.D. **(D/C)**
Cherry St.
P. O. Box 400
Leslie, AR 72645
(501) 447-2599
AC,CT,DD,IM,NT,PM,RHU

Little Rock

Norbert J. Becquet, M.D. **(DIPL)**
115 W. Sixth Street
Little Rock, AR 72201
(501) 375-4419
CT,OPH,PM,RHU

Springdale

Doty Murphy III, M.D. **(P)**
812 Dorman
Springdale, AR 72764
(501) 756-3251
CD,CT

CALIFORNIA

Albany

Ross B. Gordon, M.D. **(DIPL)**
405 Kains Avenue
Albany, CA 94706
(415) 526-3232
BA,CT,NT,PM

Auburn

Zane Kime, M.D. **(P)**
1212 High St., Ste 204
Auburn, CA 95603
(916) 823-3421
A,AR,CD,CT,NT,PM

Burbank

Douglas Hunt, M.D. **(P)**
3808 Riverside Drive
Ste 600, Penthouse
Burbank, CA 91505
(818) 840-8322
A,NT,PM

Campbell

Carol A. Shamlin, M.D. **(P)**
621 E. Campbell, Ste 11A
Campbell, CA 95008
(408) 378-7970
A,CT,GP,MM,OME,PM

Covina

James R. Privitera, M.D. **(P)**
105 Grand View
Covina, CA 91723
(818) 966-1618
A,MM,NT

Crescent City

Carl V. Lansing, M.D.
705 N. Pebble Beach
Crescent City, CA 95531
(707) 464-2144
(Retired)

Dixon

Alvin H. Gullock, M.D. **(P)**
255 N. Lincoln, Ste A
Dixon, CA 95620
(916) 678-5706
A,BA,FP

El Cajon

William J. Saccoman, M.D. **(P)**
505 N. Mollison Ave., Ste 103
El Cajon, CA 92021
(619) 440-3838
CT,NT,PM

El Toro

David A. Steenblock, D.O.
(DIPL)
22821 Lake Forest Dr., Ste 114
El Toro, CA 92630
(714) 770-9616
CD,CT,DIA,IM

Encino

Charles Canfield, M.D.
16311 Ventura Blvd. #725
Encino, CA 91436
(Retired)

A. Leonard Klepp, M.D. **(DIPL)**
16311 Ventura Blvd. #725
Encino, CA 91436
(818) 981-5511
CT,FP,PM,HGL,NT

Fresno

David J. Edwards, M.D. **(DIPL)**
360 S. Clovis Ave.
Fresno, CA 93727
(209) 251-5066
GYN,PM,CT

Hollywood

James J. Julian, M.D. **(P)**
1654 Cahuenga Blvd.
Hollywood, CA 90028
(213) 467-5555
AR,BA,CT,NT,PM

Huntington Beach

Glen C. Mahoney, M.D. **(DIPL)**
2223 Main St., Ste 44
Huntington Beach, CA 92648
(714) 969-5255
A,AR,CT,GE,NT

Robert Peterson, D.O. **(P)**
8041 Newman Ave., Ste 100
Huntington Beach, CA 92647
(714) 841-6355
AR,CD,CT,DD,FP,GP

Kentfield

Carolyn Albrecht, M.D.
10 Wolfgrade
Kentfield, CA 94904
(Retired)

Laytonville

Eugene D. Finkle, M.D. **(P)**
50 Branscomb Road
P. O. Box 309
Laytonville, CA 95454
(707) 984-6151
CT,GP,GYN,MM,NT,PM

Loma Linda

Bruce W. Halstead, M.D. **(P)**
11155 Mountain View Ave.
Suite 101
Loma Linda, CA 92354
(714) 799-3187
PM,HO,CT

Long Beach

H. Richard Casdorph, M.D.,
Ph.D. **(DIPL)**
1703 Termino Ave., Ste 201
Long Beach, CA 90804
(213) 597-8716
CD,CS,CT,DIA,IM,NT

Los Altos

Robert F. Cathcart III, M.D. **(P)**
127 Second St., Ste 4
Los Altos, CA 94022
(415) 949-2822
A,AR,CT,DD,OME,PM

Los Angeles

M. Jahangiri, M.D. **(P)**
2156 South Santa Fe
Los Angeles, CA 90058
(213) 587-3218
A,AC,CT,FP,GP

Anita Millen, M.D. **(P)**
1539 Sawtelle Blvd., Ste 10
Los Angeles, CA 90025
(213) 478-1718
CT,FP,GYN,NT,PM,DD

Monrovia

Douglas M. Baird Jr., D.O.
416 Jeffries Avenue
Space 15
Monrovia, CA 91016
(No Referrals)

C. Fred Hering III, M.D. **(P)**
212-A W. Foothill Blvd.
Monrovia, CA 91016
(818) 357-2226
CT,PM,NT

Moorpark

Ward Dean, M.D. **(P)**
12500 Arbor Hill St.
Moorpark, CA
(213) 275-9616
BA,CT,GER,NT,OS,PM

Mountain View

Claude Marquette, M.D. **(P)**
525 South Dr., Ste 115
Mountain View, CA 94040
(415) 964-6700
A,BA,CT,NT,PM

North Highlands

Garry F. Gordon, M.D. **(DIPL)**
3325 Myrtle Ave.
North Highlands, CA 95660-5154
(916) 348-4000
CT,PM,NT

North Hollywood

David Freeman, M.D. **(P)**
11311 Camarillo St. #309
N. Hollywood, CA 91602
(818) 985-1103
CD,CT,END,HGL,NT,PM

Palm Springs

David H. Tang, M.D. **(P)**
Palm Springs, CA
(415) 382-9040 (temporary)
(full address not available at
present time)
AC,CT,IM,MM,NT,PM

Petaluma

Mortimer Weiss, M.D. **(DIPL)**
1580 E. Washington
Petaluma, CA 94952
(707) 762-5533
A,AC,CT,NT,PM

Rancho Mirage

Charles Farinella, M.D. **(P)**
69-730 Hwy. 111, Ste 106A
Rancho Mirage, CA 92270
(619) 324-0734
CT,GP,PM

Red Bluff

Eva Jalkotzy, M.D. **(P)**
2150 Main St., Ste 14
Red Bluff, CA 96080
(916) 527-9182 or
(916) 527-9183
CT,FP,GP,NT,PM

Sacramento

Michael Kwiker, D.O. **(P)**
3301 Alta Arden, Ste 3
Sacramento, CA 95825
(916) 489-4400
A,CT,DIA,NT

San Diego

T. Dosumu-Johnson, M.D.
(DIPL)
5222 Balboa Ave., Ste 62
San Diego, CA 92117
(619) 492-9101
CT,GP,IM

San Francisco

Robert Haskell, M.D. **(P)**
5133 Geary Blvd.
San Francisco, CA 94118
(415) 668-1300
NT,PM

Paul Lynn, M.D. **(P)**
345 W. Portal Ave.
San Francisco, CA 94127
(415) 566-1000
A,AR,CT,DD,NT,PM

San Jose

Eddie F. Barr, M.D. **(P)**
930 Town & Country Village
San Jose, CA 95128
(408) 247-7521
CT,DIA,GP,PM

Lon B. Work, M.D. **(D/C)**
1346 Ridder Park Dr.
San Jose, CA 95232
(408) 437-1192
GYN,DD,CT,RHU,NT,HGL

San Leandro

Steven H. Gee, M.D. **(P)**
595 Estudillo St.
San Leandro, CA 94577
(415) 483-5881
AC,BA,GP

San Rafael

Robert Haskell, M.D. **(P)**
4144 Redwood Highway
San Rafael, CA 94903
(415) 499-9377
CT,NT,PM

Santa Ana

Robert B. Gold, D.O. **(P)**
1905 N. College Ave.
Suite B-2
Santa Ana, CA 92706
(714) 541-4080
BA,CT,DD,GER,NT,PM

Santa Barbara

Henry J. Hoegerman, M.D.
(DIPL)
101 W. Arrellaga
Santa Barbara, CA 93101
(805) 963-1824
A,CT,CD,GP,DIA,FP,RHU

Mohamed Moharram, M.D. **(P)**
101 W. Arrellaga, Ste B
Santa Barbara, CA 93101
(805) 965-5229
CT,CS,DIA,DD,GP,PM

Santa Cruz

Lon B. Work, M.D. **(D/C)**
1717 Seabright Ave., Ste 1
Santa Cruz, CA 95062
(408) 423-1411
GYN,DD,CT,RHU,NT,HGL

Santa Maria

Donald E. Reiner, M.D. **(P)**
1414-D South Miller
Santa Maria, CA 93454
(805) 925-0961
CT,GP,OME,PM,S

Santa Monica

Laszlo I. Belenyessy, M.D. **(P)**
2901 Wilshire Blvd., Ste 435
Santa Monica, CA 90403
(213) 828-4480
A,AC,BA,CT,GP,NT

Murray Susser, M.D. **(DIPL)**
2730 Wilshire Blvd., Ste 110
Santa Monica, CA 90403
(213) 453-4424
A,CT,NT

Seal Beach

Murray Susser, M.D. **(DIPL)**
909 Electric Ave., Ste 212
Seal Beach, CA 90740
(213) 493-4526
A,CT,NT

Sherman Oaks

Rosa M. Ami Belli, M.D.
13481 Cheltenham Dr.
Sherman Oaks, CA 91423
(No Referrals)

Wayne R. Weber, M.D. **(P)**
3235 Longridge Terrace
Sherman Oaks, CA 91423
(818) 789-4228
CT,GYN,MM,NT

Stanton

William J. Goldwag, M.D. **(P)**
7499 Cerritos Ave.
Stanton, CA 90680
(714) 827-5180
CT,NT,PM

Temecula

K. Peter McCallum, M.D. **(DIPL)**
28561 Front, Ste 9
Temecula, CA 92380
CT,NT,PM,MM,OME

Van Nuys

Frank Mosler, M.D. **(P)**
14428 Gilmore St.
Van Nuys, CA 91401
(818) 785-7425
BA,CT,GP,HGL,NT,PM

Walnut Creek

Alan Shifman Charles, M.D. **(P)**
1414 Maria Lane
Walnut Creek, CA 94596
(415) 937-3331
AC,CT,DD,FP,OME,OSM

COLORADO

Colorado Springs

James R. Fish, M.D. **(DIPL)**
3030 N. Hancock
Colorado Springs, CO 80907
(303) 471-2273
CT,HYP,PM

Denver

Edward Anderson, D.O. **(P)**
180 Adams, Ste 200
Denver, CO 80206
(303) 388-2411
A,BA,CT,NT,PM,OSM

Grand Junction

William L. Reed, M.D. **(D/C)**
591 25 Road, Ste A-4
Grand Junction, Co 81505
(303) 241-3631
AN,CT,NT,PM

Wheat Ridge

William Doell, D.O. **(DIPL)**
7777 W. 38th Ave.
Wheat Ridge, CO 80033
(303) 422-0585
AR,CT,FP,HGL,NT,OSM

CONNECTICUT

Bristol

Herbert J. Douglas, M.D. **(D/C)**
100 Franklin St.
Bristol, CT 06010
(203) 584-1931
AN,BA,CD,CS,GP,PMR

DISTRICT OF COLUMBIA

Washington

George Mitchell, M.D. **(DIPL)**
2112 F Street, N.W.
Washington, D.C. 20037
(202) 429-9456
A,CT,NT

FLORIDA

Altamonte Springs

Robert J. Rogers, M.D. **(DIPL)**
E. Altamonte Dr., Ste 304
Altamonte Springs, FL 32701
(407) 830-9355
CT,NT,PM,A,CD

Bradenton

E. Randall Horton, Jr., D.O. **(P)**
401 Manatee Ave., East
Bradenton, FL 33508
(813) 748-7943
CT,GP,HGL,NT,OSM

Chin Yong Lee, M.D. **(P)**
4301 32nd St. W., Ste C20
Bradenton, FL 34205
Office: (813) 753-6188
Answering Service:
(813) 756-8833
A,AR,AU,CT,DD,OME

C.Y. Lee Cho, M.D. **(P)**
2600 Gulf Dr., Ste 20 So.
Bradenton Bch., FL 34210
Office: (813) 753-6188
Answering Service:
(813) 756-8833
A,AR,AU,CT,DD,OME

Casselberry

Gordon S. Parsons, D.O. **(D/C)**
1120 Semoran Blvd.
Casselberry, FL 32707
(407) 678-2400
CT,FP,OSM

Crystal River

Eileen O'Ferrell Adams, M.D.
P. O. Box 820
Holiday Dr. & Hwy. 44
Crystal River, FL 32629
(Retired)

Ft. McCoy

George Graves, D.O. **(P)**
P. O. Box 2220
Ft. McCoy, FL 32637
(904) 236-2525
CT,DD,PM

Holly Hill

Sam D. Matheny, D.O. **(P)**
1722 Ridgewood Ave.
Holly Hill, FL 32017
(904) 672-2111
OSM,S

Hollywood

Herbert Pardell, D.O. **(DIPL)**
1818 Sheridan Street
Hollywood, FL 33020
(305) 922-7333
CT,DD,IM,MM,NT,PM

Richard Sabates, M.D. **(P)**
1818 Sheridan Street
Hollywood, FL 33020
(305) 922-7333
CT,FP,NT,PM

Jupiter

Neil Ahner, M.D. **(D/C)**
535 E. Indiantown Rd.
Jupiter, FL 33477
(407) 744-0077
CT,NT,PM

Lakeland

Harold Robinson, M.D. **(D/C)**
4406 S. Florida Ave., Ste 27
Lakeland, FL 33803
(813) 646-5088
CT,FP,GP,HGL,NT,PM

Lake Park

Charles E. Curtis, D.O. **(P)**
310 U.S. Highway 1
Lake Park, FL 33403
(305) 848-1623
CT,FP,OSM

Lauderdale by the Sea

Wilfred Mittelstadt, D.O. **(P)**
4001 Ocean Dr., Ste 305
Lauderdale by the Sea, FL 33308
(305) 491-4656
CT,NT,PM

Melbourne

Robert J. Rogers, M.D. **(DIPL)**
15 W. and 19 W. Ave. B
Melbourne, FL 32901
(407) 723-2360
A,CD,CT,NT,PM

Miami

Joseph G. Godorov, D.O. **(P)**
9055 S.W. 87th Ave. #307
Miami, FL 33178
(305) 595-0671
CT,END,FP,HGL,NT,PM

North Lauderdale

Narinder Singh Parhar, M.D. **(P)**
Tam O'Shanter Plaza
1333 S. State Road 7
N. Lauderdale, FL 33068
(Phone not available at present time)
GP

North Miami Beach

Martin Dayton, D.O. **(DIPL)**
18600 Collins Ave.
N. Miami Beach, FL 33160
(305) 931-8484
CT,FP,GER,NT,OSM,PM

Robert E. Willner, M.D. **(P)**
16400 N.E. 19th Avenue
N. Miami Beach, FL 33162
(305) 949-6331
BA,CT,GP

North Palm Beach

Douglas M. Baird, D.O. **(P)**
630 U.S. Highway 1, Ste 400
N. Palm Beach, FL 33408
(407) 844-6363
CT,DD

Ocala

Sheldon Katanick, D.O. **(P)**
3405 S.W. College Road
Orlando, FL 32674
(904) 237-4133
P,NT,Radiology

Orlando

Joya Lynn Schoen, M.D. **(P)**
1900 N. Orange Ave.
Orlando, FL 32804
(407) 898-2951
A,CT,HGL,OSM,Homeopathy

Pompano Beach

Dan C. Roehm, M.D. **(D/C)**
3400 Park Central Blvd., North
Suite 3450
Pompano Beach, FL 33064
(305) 977-3700
CD,CT,IM,MM,NT,OME

Royal Palm Beach

Domenico Caporusso, M.D.
(D/C)
11476 Okeechobee Blvd.
Royal Palm Beach, FL 33411
(407) 793-7548
BA,CT,FP,NT,PM

St. Petersburg

Ray Wunderlich Jr., M.D. **(D/C)**
666 6th St., South
St. Petersburg, FL 33408
(813) 822-3612
A,BA,CT,DD,HGL,MM,PO

Tampa

Donald J. Carrow, M.D. **(P)**
4525 S. Manhattan Ave.
Tampa, FL 33611
(813) 832-3220
AR,CD,DIA,HGL,HO

Eugene H. Lee, M.D. **(P)**
305 S. Brevard, Ste 1
Tampa, FL 33606
(813) 251-3089
AC,CT,NT,PM,GP,HGL

Wauchula

Alfred S. Massam, M.D. **(P)**
528 West Main St.
P. O. Box 1328
Wauchula, FL 33873
(813) 773-6668
CT,FP,PM

Winterhaven

Russell B. Hays, M.D.
P. O. Box 9205
1556 6th St., S.E.
Winterhaven, FL 33880
(Retired)

GEORGIA

Atlanta

Milton Fried, M.D. **(D/C)**
4426 Tilly Mill Rd.
Atlanta, GA 30360
(404) 451-4857
A,IM,NT,PM,CT,PO

Camilla

Oliver L. Gunter, M.D. **(D/C)**
P. O. Box 347
24 N. Ellis St.
Camilla, GA 31730
(912) 336-7343
CT,DIA,DD,GP,NT,PUD

Norcross

Bernard Mlaver, M.D. **(D/C)**
3700 Holcomb Bridge Rd., Ste 6
Norcross, GA 300921
(404) 448-4535
CT,NT,PM

Warner Robins

Terril J. Schneider, M.D. **(P)**
205 Dental Dr., Ste 3
Warner Robins, GA 31088
(912) 929-1027
A,CT,FP,NT,PM,PMR

HAWAII

Honolulu

Richard Renn, D.O. **(P)**
1481 S. King St., Ste 539
Honolulu, HI 96814
(808) 941-0522
CT,NT,PM

Kailua-Kona

Clifton Arrington, M.D. **(P)**
P. O. Box 649
Kealakekua-Kona, HI 96750
(808) 322-9400
BA,CT,FP,NT,PM

IDAHO

Coeur d'Alene

Charles T. McGee, M.D. **(P)**
1717 Lincolnway, Ste 108
Coeur d'Alene, ID 83814
(208) 664-1478
A,CT,NT,OME,PM

Nampa

John O. Boxall, M.D. **(P)**
824 117th Ave., South
Nampa, ID 83651
(208) 466-3518
AC,CT,GP,HYP

ILLINOIS

Arlington Heights

Cassim Igram, D.O. **(P)**
3345 N. Arlington Heights Rd.,
Ste D
Arlington Heights, IL 60004
(312) 577-5252
A,BA,CT,DD,NT,PM

William Mauer, D.O. **(DIPL)**
3401 N. Kennicott Ave.
Arlington Heights, IL 60003
(312) 255-8988
CT,FP,HGL,NT,OSM

Belvidere

M. Paul Dommers, M.D. **(D/C)**
554 S. Main Street
Belvidere, IL 61008
(815) 544-3112
AR,AU,CT,MM,PM

Chicago

Razvan Rentea, M.D. **(P)**
3354 N. Paulina
Chicago, IL 60657
(312) 549-0101
GP,MM,PM

Coal Valley

Gary L. Pynckel, D.O. **(DIPL)**
201 W. 2nd Ave.
Coal Valley, IL 61240
(309) 799-7301
CT,FP,GP,OSM,PM

Glen Ellyn

Robert S. Waters, M.D. **(DIPL)**
739 Roosevelt Rd.
Bldg. 8, Ste 314
Glen Ellyn, IL 60137
(312) 790-8100
CT,PM,OME

Homewood

Frederick Weiss, M.D.
3207 W. 184th Street
Homewood, IL 60430
(No Referrals)

Maryville

Tipu Sultan, M.D. **(P)**
1050 N. Center
Maryville, IL 62062
(618) 288-3233
A,AR,CT,HGL,PM

Metamora

Stephen K. Elsasser, D.O. **(DIPL)**
205 S. Engelwood
Metamora, IL 61548
(309) 367-2321
CT,GP,HO,NT,OSM,PM

Ottawa

Terry W. Love, D.O. **(D/C)**
P. O. Box 547
Ottawa, IL 61350-0547
AR,CT,GP,OSM,PM,RHU

Palatine

Terrill K. Haws, D.O. **(D/C)**
1542 N. Norway Lane, Ste 1A
Palatine, IL 60067
(312) 577-9451
CT,DD,FP,GP,OSM

Woodstock

John R. Tambone, M.D. **(P)**
102 E. South Street
Woodstock, IL 60098
(815) 338-2345
A,CT,GP,HYP,NT,PM

INDIANA

Clarksville

George Wolverton, M.D. **(DIPL)**
647 Eastern Blvd.
Clarksville, IN 47130
(812) 282-4309
CD,CT,FP,GYN,PD,PM

Evansville

Harold T. Sparks, D.O. **(P)**
3001 Washington Ave.
Evansville, IN 47714
(812) 479-8228
A,AC,BA,CT,FP,PM

Highland

Cal Streeter, D.O. **(P)**
9635 Saric Court
Highland, IN 46322
(219) 924-2410
A,CD,CT,FP,OSM,PM

Indianapolis

David A. Darbro, M.D. **(DIPL)**
2124 E. Hanna Ave.
Indianapolis, IN 46227
(317) 787-7221
A,AR,CT,DD,FP,PM

Mooresville

Norman E. Whitney, D.O. **(P)**
P. O. Box 173
Mooresville, IN 46158
(317) 831-3352
AR,CD,DD,DIA,FP,NT

South Bend

David E. Turfler, D.O. **(P)**
336 W. Navarre St.
South Bend, IN 46616
(219) 233-3840
A,FP,GP,HGL,OBS,OSM

KANSAS

Garden City

Terry Hunsberger, D.O. **(P)**
602 N. 3rd
P. O. Box 679
Garden City, KS 67846
(316) 275-7128
BA,CT,FP,NT,OSM,PM

Hays

Roy N. Neil, M.D. **(P)**
105 West 13th
Hays, KS 67601
(913) 628-8341
BA,CD,CT,DD,NT,PM

Wichita

Stevens B. Acker, M.D. **(DIPL)**
1100 N. St. Francis, Ste 400
Wichita, KS 67214
(316) 263-7002
CT,DD,FP,MM,PM

KENTUCKY

Bowling Green

John C. Tapp, M.D. **(D/C)**
414 Old Morgantown Rd.
Bowling Green, KY 42101
(502) 781-1483
CT,GYN,MM,PD,P,RHU

Lexington

Walt Stoll, M.D. **(P)**
1412 N. Broadway, Ste 207
Lexington, KY 40505
(606) 233-4273
CT,FP,NT,PM

Louisville

Kirk Morgan, M.D. **(DIPL)**
9105 U.S. Hwy. 42
Louisville, KY 40059
(502) 228-0156
CT,FP

LOUISIANA

Baton Rouge

Steve Kuplesky, M.D. **(DIPL)**
7324 Alberta Dr.
Baton Rouge, LA 70808
(504) 769-8503
FP,MM,NT

Bossier City

James R. Bruner, M.D. **(P)**
2225 Beckett St.
Bossier City, LA 71111
(318) 747-7121
BA,CD,CT,S

Chalmette

Saroj T. Tampira, M.D. **(P)**
812 E. Judge Perez
Chalmette, LA 70043
(504) 277-8991
CD,CT,DD,DIA,IM

Harahan

James M. Foster, M.D. **(P)**
2020 Dickory, Ste 100
Harahan, LA 70123
(504) 733-1100
AR,GER,HO,PM,CT,NT
Environmental Medicine

Mandeville

Roy M. Montalbano, M.D. **(P)**
4408 Highway 22
Mandeville, LA 70448
(504) 626-1985
CT,FP,NT,PM

Newellton

Joseph R. Whitaker, M.D. **(P)**
P. O. Box 458
Newellton, LA 71357
(318) 467-5731
CT,GP,IM

New Iberia

Adonis J. Domingue, M.D. **(D/C)**
222 Weeks Street
New Iberia, LA 70560
(318) 365-2196
GP

New Orleans

James P. Carter, M.D. **(P)**
1430 Tulane Avenue
New Orleans, LA 70112
(504) 588-5136
GP,NT,PM,CT

Shreveport

James R. Bruner, M.D. **(P)**
P. O. Box 18097
9435 Mansfield Rd., Ste 1B
Shreveport, LA 71082
(318) 687-3100

R. Denman Crow, M.D. **(P)**
1545 Line Ave., Ste 222
Shreveport, LA 71101-4669
(318) 221-1569
A,FP,GP,GYN,PM,PUD

MARYLAND

Laurel

Paul V. Beals, M.D. **(D/C)**
9101 Cherry Ln Park, Ste 205
Laurel, MD 20708
(301) 490-9911
CT,FP,NT,PM

MASSACHUSETTS

Cambridge

Michael Janson, M.D. **(P)**
2557 Massachusetts Ave.
Cambridge, MA 02140
(617) 661-6225
CT,IM,OME,PM

Newton Centre

Carol Englender, M.D. **(P)**
1340 Centre Street
Newton Centre, MA 02159
(617) 965-7770
A,FP,NT,PM,Env.Medicine

Westfield

Vincent A. Longobardo, M.D.
(D/C)
Westfield Executive Park
53 S. Hampton Road
Westfield, MA 01085
(413) 562-7539 or
(413) 562-7530
AN,BA,CT

MICHIGAN

Atlanta

Leo Modzinsky, D.O., M.D. **(P)**
100 W. State Street
Atlanta, MI 49709
(517) 785-4254
BA,CT,FP,GP,NT,OSM

Bay City

Doyle B. Hill, D.O. **(D/C)**
907 Cass Avenue
Bay City, MI 48706
(517) 892-3549
A,CT,FP,GP,NT,OSM

Doyle B. Hill, D.O. **(D/C)**
2520 Euclid Ave.
Bay City, MI 48706
(517) 686-5200
A,CT,FP,GP,NT,OSM

David M. Mac, D.O. **(P)**
G-3479 Fenton Rd.
Burton, MI 48529
(313) 234-1697
CT,FP,NT,PM,OBS,S

Detroit

John Barkay, D.O. **(P)**
13850 East 8 Mile Rd.
Detroit, MI 48205
(313) 371-0044
CT,FP,PM,OME,OSM

Richard E. Tapert, D.O. **(DIPL)**
15850 E. Warren Ave.
Detroit, MI 48224
(313) 885-5405
CT,GP,NT,PM

Farmington Hills

Paul A. Parente, D.O. **(P)**
29538 Orchard Lake Rd.
Farmington Hills, MI 48018
(313) 626-7544
BA,CT,GP,PM

Paul A. Parente, D.O. **(P)**
30275 Thirteen Mile Rd.
Farmington Hills, MI 48018
(313) 626-9690
BA,CT,GP,PM

Albert J. Scarchilli, D.O. **(DIPL)**
29538 Orchard Lake Rd.
Farmington Hills, MI 48018
(313) 626-7544
BA,CT,FP,GP,MM,OSM,PM

Albert Scarchilli, D.O.
30275 Thirteen Mile Rd.
Farmington Hills, MI 48018
(313) 626-9690
BA,CT,FP,GP,MM,OSM,PM

Flint

William M. Bernard, D.O. **(P)**
1044 Gilbert Street
Flint, MI 48532
(313) 733-3140
A,CT,FP,GER,OSM,PM

Kurt W. Mikat, M.D. **(P)**
401 S. Ballenger Hwy.
Flint, MI 48532-3685
(313) 762-2197
Pathology

Grand Haven

E. Duane Powers, D.O.
P. O. Box 170
Grand Haven, MI 49417
(Retired)

Grand Rapids

Grant Born, D.O. **(DIPL)**
2687 44th St., SE
Grand Rapids, MI 49508
(616) 455-3550
A,CT,FP,GYN,PM,PMR

James Nutt, D.O. **(P)**
2730 5 Mile Road, NE
Grand Rapids, MI 49505
(616) 361-5000
A,AC,CT,GER,BA,PM

Greenville

James Nutt, D.O. **(P)**
420 South Lafayette
Greenville, MI 48838
(616) 754-3679
A,AC,BA,CT,GER,PM

Linden

Marvin D. Penwell, D.O. **(D/C)**
319 S. Bridge St.
Linden, MI 48451
(313) 735-7809
A,CT,FP,GE,GYN,OSM

Pontiac

Vahagn Agbabian, D.O. **(P)**
28 North Saginaw St. #1105
Pontiac, MI 48058-3390
(313) 334-2424
CT,DD,DIA,GER,IM,OME

Southgate

Ole C. Kistler, D.O.
12100 Dix-Toledo Rd.
Southgate, MI 48195
(313) 285-2620
CT,GP,OSM

Williamston

Seldon R. Nelson, D.O. **(P)**
4386 N. Meridian Road
Williamston, MI 48895
(517) 349-5346
AR,CT,GP,NT,OSM

MINNESOTA

Plymouth

Jean R. Eckerly, M.D. **(DIPL)**
Preventive Medical Association
10700 Old Country Rd. 15
Suite 350
Plymouth, MN 55441
(612) 593-9458
CT,IM,NT,OME,PM

Judith Lewis, D.O. **(D/C)**
Preventive Medical Association
10700 Old Country Rd. 15
Suite 350
Plymouth, MN 55441
(612) 593-9458
OSM

MISSISSIPPI

Coldwater

Pravinchandra Patel, M.D. **(P)**
P. O. Drawer DD
Coldwater, MS 38618-0924
(601) 736-2376
CT,FP

Ocean Springs

James H. Waddell, M.D. **(D/C)**
1112 La Fontaine St.
Ocean Springs, MS 39564
(601) 875-5441
AC,AN,AU,CT

Shelby

Robert T. Hollingsworth, M.D. **(DIPL)**
Drawer 87, 901 Forrest St.
Shelby, MS 38774
(601) 398-5106
CT,FP,GYN,OSB,PD,S

MISSOURI

Excelsior Springs

Albert Leo Pfauth, D.O. **(P)**
102 Collette St.
Excelsior Springs, MO 64024
(816) 637-6188
CT,GP,NT

Festus

John T. Schwent, D.O. **(P)**
1400 Truman Blvd.
Festus, MO 63028
(314) 937-8688
A,CT,FP,NT,OBS,OSM

Florissant

Tipu Sultan, M.D. **(P)**
4585 Washington St.
Florissant, MO 63033
(314) 921-7100
A,AR,CT,HGL,PM

Independence

Lawrence E. Dorman, D.O. **(P)**
9120 E. 35th Street
Independence, MO 64052
(816) 358-2712
AC,CT,MM,OSM,PM

James E. Swann, D.O. **(DIPL)**
2116 Sterling
Independence, MO 64052
(816) 833-3366
CD,CT,DD,FP,IM,S

Jamesport

F. B. Bailey, D.O. **(P)**
Box 232
Jamesport, MO 64648
(816) 684-6614
CT,GP,OSM

Kansas City

Edward W. McDonagh, D.O. **(DIPL)**
2800-A Kendallwood Pkwy.
Kansas City, MO 64119
(816) 453-5940
CD,CT,DD,FP,HO,PM

James Rowland, D.O. **(P)**
8133 Wornall Road
Kansas City, MO 64114
(816) 361-4077
AC,CT,DD,GP,HYP,OSM

Charles J. Rudolph, D.O., Ph.D., **(DIPL)**
2800-A Kendallwood Pkwy.
Kansas City, MO 64119
(816) 453-5940
CD,CT,DD,FP,HO,PM

Raytown

Kenneth Adler, D.O. **(P)**
10007 E. 66th Terrace
Raytown, MO 64133
(816) 353-3050 or
(816) 353-3051
CT,GP,OSM

Salem

Bob R. Carnett, D.O. **(P)**
P. O. Box 40
Rolla Rd. at McArthur St.
Salem, MO 65560
(314) 729-6225
CT,FP,OSM,PM

Springfield

William C. Sunderwirth, D.O.
(P)
2828 N. National
Springfield, MO 65803
(417) 869-6260
CT,DIA,GP,OSM,PM,S

William C. Sunderwirth, D.O.
(P)
307 South Street
Springfield, MO 65803
(417) 276-3221
CT,DIA,GP,OSM,PM,S

G. Fred Warren, D.O. **(P)**
604 South Pickwick
Springfield, MO 65802
(417) 864-5986
GP,NT,CT,PM

St. Louis

Heyden Hucke, M.D. **(D/C)**
23 N. Gore
St. Louis, MO 63119
(314) 961-6631
CT,FP,GER,GYN,NT,PM

Harvey Walker Jr., M.D., Ph.D.
(DIPL)
138 N. Meramec Ave.
St. Louis, MO 63105
(314) 721-7227
CT,DIA,HGL,IM,NT,PM

Sullivan

Ronald H. Scott, D.O. **(P)**
131 Meredith Lane
Sullivan, MO 63080
(314) 468-4932
GP,GER,GYN,NT,PM,OSM

MONTANA

Whitefish

David V. Kauffman, M.D. **(DIPL)**
P. O. Box 1837
Whitefish, MT 59937-1837
(406) 862-3961
CT,FP,GYN,HGL,OBS,PD

NEVADA

Las Vegas

Robert D. Milne, M.D. **(P)**
501 S. Rancho, Ste 44G
Las Vegas, NV 89106
(702) 385-1999
A,AC,CT,FP,NT,PM

Robert Vance, D.O. **(DIPL)**
801 S. Rancho Dr. #F-2
Las Vegas, NV 89106
(702) 385-7771
A,CT,HO,MM,OSM,PM

Reno

Michael L. Gerber, M.D. **(DIPL)**
3670 Grant Drive
Reno, NV 89509
(702) 826-1900
CT,MM,OME

Donald E. Soli, M.D. **(P)**
19 Winter Street
Reno, NV 89503
(702) 786-7101
A,AR,CT,HGL,HO,PUD

Yiwen Y. Tang, M.D. **(P)**
380 Brinkby
Reno, NV 89509
(702) 826-9500
A,CD,CT,HGL,HO,PM

NEW JERSEY

Edison

Ralph Lev, M.D., M.S. **(DIPL)**
952 Amboy Avenue
Edison, NJ 08837
(201) 738-9220
CD,CT,S

Marlton

Allan Magaziner, D.O. **(D/C)**
8002-A Greentree Commons
Marlton, NJ 08053
(609) 596-3030
CT,NT,OSM,PM,
Environmental Medicine

Paramus

Linda Choi, M.D. **(P)**
585 Winters Ave.
Paramus, NJ 07652
(201) 967-5081
CT,GP,NT,PM

James Turner, M.D. **(D/C)**
585 Winters Ave.
Paramus, NJ 07652
(201) 967-5081
GP

West Orange

Faina Munits, M.D., Ph.D. **(D/C)**
51 Pleasant Valley Way
West Orange, NJ 07052
(201) 736-3743
A,CD,DIA,DD,HGL,PM

NEW MEXICO

Albuquerque

Fred R. Holzworth, M.D. **(P)**
4101 Montgomery Blvd., N.E.
Albuquerque, NM 87109
(505) 883-1233
BA,CT,HGL,PM,RHU

Gerald Parker, D.O. **(P)**
6208 Montgomery
Albuquerque, NM 87109
(505) 884-3506
A,CT,AC,AR,GP,HO

John T. Taylor, D.O. **(P)**
6208 Montgomery
Albuquerque, NM 87110
(505) 884-3506
A,CT,AC,AR,GP,HO

Paul Wynn, D.O. **(P)**
4101 Montgomery Blvd., N.E.
Albuquerque, NM 87109
(505) 883-1233
BA,CT,PM

Clovis

Gerald Parker, D.O. **(P)**
309 Main
Clovis, NM 88102
(505) 769-1014
A,AC,AR,CT,GP,HO ·

John T. Taylor, D.O. **(P)**
309 Main
Clovis, NM 88102
(505) 769-1014
A,AC,AR,CT,GP,HO

Portales

E. L. Miller, D.O. **(D/C)**
401 S. Avenue, Ste A
Portales, NM 88130
(505) 356-4471
CT,GER,GP

Roswell

Annette Stoesser, M.D. **(D/C)**
112 S. Kentucky
Roswell, NM 88201
(505) 623-2444
A,CT,DIA,DD,FP,NT

NEW YORK

Falconer

Reino F. Hill, M.D. **(P)**
230 West Main St.
Falconer, NY 14733
(716) 665-3505
CT,FP,PM

Huntington

Serafina Corsello, M.D. **(DIPL)**
175 E. Main Street
Huntington, NY 11743
(516) 271-0222
CT,DD,MM,NT,OME,PM

Lawrence

Mitchell Kurk, M.D. **(P)**
310 Broadway
Lawrence, NY 11559
(516) 239-5540
CT,FP,GER,NT,OME,PM

New York

Robert C. Atkins, M.D.
(DIPL)
400 East 56th Street
New York, NY 10022
(212) 758-2110
CT,HGL,OME

Serafina Corsello, M.D. **(DIPL)**
34 East 67th Street
New York, NY 10021
(212) 517-2222
CT,DD,MM,NT,OME,PM

Ronald Hoffman, M.D. **(P)**
125 West 87th Street
New York, NY 10024
(212) 496-5482
A,FP,HGL,NT,PM

Richard Izquierodo, M.D. **(P)**
1057 Southern Blvd.
New York, NY 10452
(212) 589-4541
A,FP,GP,NT,PD,PM

Warren M. Levin, M.D. **(DIPL)**
444 Park Ave. South/30th St.
New York, NY 10016
(212) 696-1900
A,AC,CT,NT,OME,PM

Stanley H. Title, M.D. **(P)**
171 West 57th Street
New York, NY 10019
(212) 581-9532
BA,MM,NT

Nyack

Michael Schachter, M.D. **(DIPL)**
43B Route 59
Nyack, NY 10960
(914) 358-6800
A,CT,NT,PO

Orangeburg

Neil L. Block, M.D. **(P)**
14 Prell Plaza
Orangeburg, NY 10962
(914) 359-3300
A,CD,FP,IM,NT,PO

Rhinebeck

Kenneth A. Bock, M.D. **(DIPL)**
108 Montgomery St.
Rhinebeck, NY 12572
(914) 876-7082
A,CD,CT,FP,NT,PM

Watervliet

Rodolfo T. Sy, M.D. **(P)**
1845 6th Avenue
Watervliet, NY 12189
(518) 273-1325
GP,PMR

Westbury

Savely Yurkovsky, M.D. **(D/C)**
309 Medicine St.
Westbury, NY 11590
(516) 333-2929
A,CD,CS,CT,NT,PM

NORTH CAROLINA

Aberdeen

Keith Johnson, M.D. **(P)**
407 Johnson Street
Aberdeen, NC 28315
(919) 944-3267
DD,GP,GER,NT,PM,PMR

NORTH DAKOTA

Grand Forks

Richard H. Leigh, M.D. **(P)**
1600 University Ave.
Grand Forks, ND 58201
(701) 775-5527
CT,GYN,MM,NT

Minot

Brian E. Briggs, M.D. **(D/C)**
718 6th Street, S.W.
Minot, ND 58701
(701) 838-6011
CT,FP,NT

OHIO

Akron

Josephine Aronica, M.D. **(P)**
1867 W. Market Street
Akron, OH 44313
(216) 867-7361
AC,CT,NT

Bluffton

L. Terry Chappell, M.D. **(DIPL)**
122 Thurman Street
Bluffton, OH 45817
(419) 358-4627
AU,CT,FP,HYP,NT,PMR

Canton

Jack E. Slingluff, D.O. **(DIPL)**
5850 Fulton Rd., N.W.
Canton, OH 44718
(216) 494-8641
CD,CT,FP,HGL,MM,NT

Cincinnati

Kaushal K. Bhardwaj, M.D. **(P)**
8325 Colerain Ave.
Cincinnati, OH 45239
(513) 741-7467
AC,AU,CD,CS,IM,PMR

Cleveland

John M. Baron, D.O. **(P)**
4807 Rockside, Ste 100
Cleveland, OH 44131
(216) 642-0082
CT,NT,PO

James P. Frackelton, M.D. **(DIPL)**
24700 Center Ridge Rd.
Cleveland, OH 44145
(216) 835-0104
CT,HO,NT,PM

Derrick Lonsdale, M.D. **(DIPL)**
24700 Center Ridge Rd.
Cleveland, OH 44145
(216) 835-0104
NT,PM,PD

Columbus

Robert R. Hershner, D.O. **(P)**
1571 E. Livingston Ave.
Columbus, OH 43255
(614) 253-8733
FP,GP,GYN,IM,P,PD

William C. Schmelzer, M.D.
(D/C)
3520 Snouffer Road
Columbus, OH 43235
(614) 761-0555
CT,FP,GP,HYP,NT,OSM

Harold J. Wilson, M.D. **(DIPL)**
28 W. Henderson Rd.
Columbus, OH 43214
(614) 261-0151
CT,END,GP
(Retired)

Dayton

David D. Goldberg, D.O. **(DIPL)**
4444 N. Main St.
Dayton, OH 45405
(513) 277-1722
CT,GP,OSM,PM

Hubbard

James Dambrogio, D.O. **(DIPL)**
212 N. Main Street
Hubbard, OH 44425
(216) 534-9737
A,CT,GP

Paulding

Don K. Snyder, M.D. **(P)**
Route 2
Box 1271
Paulding, OH 45879
(419) 399-2045
CT,FP

Wright-Patterson AFB

Ralph J. Luciani, D.O. **(D/C)**
ASD/AESA
Wright-Patterson AFB, OH 45433
(513) 255-5822
AC,AU,FP,OSM,PM,PMR

Youngstown

James Ventresco Jr., D.O. **(P)**
3848 Tippecanoe Road
Youngstown, OH 44511
(216) 792-2349
CT,FP,NT,OSM,RHU

OKLAHOMA

Bethany

Jerald M. Gilbert, M.D. **(DIPL)**
7530 N.W. 23rd
Bethany, OK 73013
(405) 787-8550
A,CT,FP,HO,NT,PM

Edmond

Vicki J. Conrad, M.D. **(D/C)**
1616 S. Boulevard
Edmond, OK 73013
(405) 341-5691
A,CT,GP,HGL,NT,PM

Henryetta

Brent Wade Davis, D.O. **(P)**
121 South Fifth Street
Henryetta, OK 74437
(918) 652-3337
CT,FP,NT

Jenks

Leon Anderson, D.O. **(DIPL)**
121 Second Street
Jenks, OK 74037
(918) 299-5038
CT,NT,OSM

Oklahoma City

James W. Hogin, D.O. **(P)**
937 S.W. 89th, Ste C
Oklahoma City, OK 73139
(405) 631-0524
CP,CS,GE,IM,NT,OSM

Charles H. Farr, M.D., Ph.D.,
(DIPL)
8524 S. Western, Ste 107
Oklahoma City, OK 73139
(405) 752-0070
A,CT,NT,PM

Wynnewood

John Geiger, D.O. **(DIPL)**
111 Jameson Drive
P. O. Box 99
Wynnewood, OK 73098
(405) 665-2084
AU,CT,DD,FP,OSM,PM

OREGON

Eugene

John Gambee, M.D. **(P)**
66 Club Road, Ste 140
Eugene, OR 97401
(503) 686-2536
A,BA,CT,PM

Grants Pass

James Wm. Fitzsimmons Jr., M.D.
(D/C)
591 Hidden Valley Road
Grants Pass, OR 97527
(503) 474-2166
A,CT

Salem

Terence Howe Young, M.D. **(P)**
21 Oaks, Ste 240
525 Glencreek Rd., N.W.
Salem, OR 97304
(503) 371-1558
A,CT,GP,OSM,PM

PENNSYLVANIA

Allentown

Frederick Burton, M.D. **(D/C)**
321 E. Emmaus Ave.
Allentown, PA 18103
(215) 791-2453
CT,IM,NT,PM

Robert H. Schmidt, D.O. **(P)**
Medical Plaza Bldg.
451 Chew St., Ste 409
Allentown, PA 18102
(215) 821-2813
CT,FP,NT,PM

D. Erik Von Kiel, D.O. **(P)**
Medical Plaza Bldg.
451 Chew St., Ste 409
Allentown, PA 18102
(215) 821-2813
CT,FP,MM,NT,OSM

Bangor

Francis J. Cinelli, D.O. **(P)**
153 N. 11th Street
Bangor, PA 18013
(215) 588-4502
CT,GP,HYP

Elizabethtown

Harold C. Walmer, D.O. **(DIPL)**
50 North Market St.
Elizabethtown, PA 17022
(717) 367-1345
AC,CT,NT,OSM,PM

Greensburg

Ralph A. Miranda, M.D. **(DIPL)**
Box 108
RD #12
Greensburg, PA 15601
(412) 838-7632
CT,FP,NT,OME,PM

Hazleton

Arthur L. Koch, D.O. **(DIPL)**
57 West Juniper St.
Hazleton, PA 18201
(717) 455-4747
CT,GP,PM

Mertztown

Conrad G. Maulfair Jr., D.O.
(DIPL)
Box 71
Main Street
Mertztown, PA 19539
(215) 682-2104
A,CT,HGL

New Castle

James S. Lapcevic, D.O. **(D/C)**
Box 546
RD #6
New Castle, PA 16101-9426
(412) 924-2181
A,CT,GP,NT,OSM,S

North Versailles

Mamduh F. El-Attrache, M.D. **(P)**
215 Crooked Run Road
North Versailles, PA 15137
(412) 673-3900
BA,CT,DIA,GER,OBS,PO

Philadelphia

Lloyd Grumbles, M.D. **(DIPL)**
1528 Walnut St., Ste 1600
Philadelphia, PA 19102
(215) 790-9970
A,CT,PM

P. Jayalakshmi, M.D. **(DIPL)**
6366 Sherwood Road
Philadelphia, PA 19151
(215) 473-4226
A,AC,AR,BA,CT,DIA,DD

Joel C. Podell, D.O. **(P)**
1544 E. Cheltenham Ave.
Philadelphia, PA 19124
(215) 743-2573
A,BA,FP,HGL,NT,PM

K. R. Sampathachar, M.D.
(DIPL)
6366 Sherwood Road
Philadelphia, PA 19151
(215) 473-4226
AC,AN,CT,DD,HYP,NT

Lance Wright, M.D. **(P)**
3901 Market Street
Philadelphia, PA 19104
(215) 387-1200
DD,END,HYP,NT,PM,PO

Pittsburgh

Howard T. Lewis, M.D. **(P)**
1241 Peermont Ave.
Pittsburgh, PA 15216
(412) 531-1222
BA,CT,HGL,NT,PM

Quakertown

Harold Buttram, M.D. **(DIPL)**
RD #3
Clymer Road
Quakertown, PA 18951
(215) 536-1890
A,CT,FP,NT

Washington

Milan J. Packovich, M.D. **(DIPL)**
90 W. Chestnut Street
Washington, PA 15301
(412) 225-0300
BA,CT,IM,MM,HGL,NT

SOUTH CAROLINA

Landrum

Theodore C. Rozema, M.D.
(DIPL)
1000 E. Rutherford Rd.
Landrum, SC 29356
(803) 457-414
(800) 922-5821 (SC)
(800) 992-8350 (NAT)
CT,FP,NT,PM

Myrtle Beach

Theodore C. Rozema, M.D.
(DIPL)
4711 Highway 17
Myrtle Beach, SC 29577
(803) 293-4141
CT,FP,NT,PM

TENNESSEE

Cleveland

Maurice S. Goldman, M.D. **(P)**
2850 Westside Dr., Ste K
Cleveland, TN 37311
(615) 476-6578
CD,CS,IM

Morristown

Donald Thompson, M.D. **(P)**
P. O. Box 2088
Morristown, TN 37816
(615) 581-6367
CT,FP,GER,GP,NT,PM

TEXAS

Abilene

William Irby Fox, M.D. **(P)**
1227 N. Mockingbird Lane
Abilene, TX 79603
(915) 672-7863
CT,DIA,GP,GER,PMS,S

Alamo

Herbert Carr, D.O. **(P)**
P. O. Box 1179
Alamo, TX 78516
(512) 787-6668
CT,OSM,PM

Amarillo

Gerald Parker, D.O. **(P)**
4714 S. Western
Amarillo, TX 79109
(806) 355-8263
A,AC,AR,CT,GP,HO

John T. Taylor, D.O. **(P)**
4714 S. Western
Amarillo, TX 79109
(806) 355-8263
A,AC,AR,CT,GP,HO

Austin

William W. Halcomb, D.O. **(P)**
8311 Shoal Creek Blvd.
Austin, TX 78758
(512) 451-8149
A,CT,GP,HO,OSM,PM

Dallas

Jack R. Vinson, D.O. **(P)**
2755 Valwood Pkwy., Ste A
Dallas, TX 75234
(214) 243-7711
A,CT,NT

J. Robert Winslow, D.O. **(P)**
2745 Valwood Pkwy.
Dallas, TX 75234
(214) 241-4614
A,CD,CT,END,PM,R

El Paso

Edward J. Ettl, M.D. **(P)**
3500 North Piedras
P. O. Box 31397
El Paso, TX 79931
(915) 566-9361
AC,CT,IM,Pathology

Houston

Robert Battle, M.D. **(DIPL)**
9910 Long Point
Houston, TX 77055
(713) 932-0552
A,BA,CD,CT,FP,HGL

Jerome L. Borochoff, M.D. **(P)**
8830 Long Point, Ste 504
Houston, TX 77055
(713) 461-7517
CD,CT,FP,HO,PM

Luis E. Guerrero, M.D. **(D/C)**
2055 S. Gessner, Ste 150
Houston, TX 77063
(713) 789-0133
AC,CT,FP,NT,PM,PO

Paul McGuff, M.D., Ph.D.
(DIPL)
3838 Hillcroft, Ste 415
Houston, TX 77057
(713) 780-7019
CD,CT,GER,PM

Vladimir Rizov, M.D. **(P)**
6550 Tarnef, Ste 4
Houston, TX 77071
(713) 771-5506
AR,CT,DD,DIA,GP,IM

Humble

John Parks Trowbridge, M.D.
(DIPL)
9816 Memorial Blvd., Ste 205
Humble, TX 77338
(713) 540-2329
CT,NT,PM

Kirbyville

John L. Sessions, D.O. **(DIPL)**
1609 South Margaret
Kirbyville, TX 75956
(409)423-2166
CT,IM,OSM

Midland

Edison McCullough, M.D. **(P)**
1415 N. Big Spring St.
Midland, TX 79701
(915) 684-5161
AC,CD,CT,DD,IM,RHU

Plano

Linda Martin Ernst, D.O. **(P)**
3920 Alma Drive
Plano, TX 75023
(214) 578-1724
CT,GP,NT,PM

San Antonio

Jim P. Archer, D.O. **(P)**
4242 Medical Dr., Ste 7150
San Antonia, TX 78229
(512) 694-4091
A,CT,HO,NT,PM

Edmond Scavone, M.D.
3130 Manila
San Antonio, TX 78217
(Retired)

Webster

Ronald M. Davis, M.D. **(P)**
16932 Hwy. 3
Webster, TX 77598
(713) 338-1889
CT,GP,PM

Wichita Falls

Thomas R. Humphrey, M.D. **(P)**
2400 Rushing
Wichita Falls, TX 76308
(817) 766-4329
BA,FP,GP,HYP

VERMONT

Essex Junction

Charles Anderson, M.D. **(P)**
175 Pearl Street
P. O. Box 418
Essex Junction, VT 05452
(802) 879-6544
A,FP,GYN,MM,NT,PM

VIRGINIA

Annandale

Sohini Patel, M.D. **(P)**
7023 Little River Tnpk.
Suite 207
Annandale, VA 22003
(703) 941-3606
A,CT,NT,PM

Hinton

Harold Huffman, M.D. **(P)**
P. O. Box 155
Hinton, VA 22831
(703) 867-5242
CT,FP,PM

Norfolk

Vincent Speckhart, M.D. **(D/C)**
902 Graydon Avenue
Norfolk, VA 23507
(804) 622-0014
IM, Medical Oncology

Trout Dale

Elmer M. Cranton, M.D. **(DIPL)**
Ripshin Road
Box 44
Trout Dale, VA 24378
(703) 677-3631
A,CD,CT,FP,HO,NT

WASHINGTON

Bellingham

Robert Kimmel, M.D. **(P)**
1800 C St., Ste C-8
Bellingham, WA 98225
(206) 734-3250
AC,CT,DD,FP,NT,PM

Kent

Sandra C. Denton, M.D. **(DIPL)**
24030 132nd Ave., S.E.
Kent, WA 98042
(206) 631-8920
CT,NT,PM,Emergency Medicine
Environmental Medicine

Maurice L. Stephens, M.D. **(D/C)**
24030 132nd Ave., S.E.
Kent, WA 98042
(206) 631-8920
CT,NT,PM
Environmental Medicine

Kirkland

Jonathan Collin, M.D. **(DIPL)**
12911 128th St., N.E.
Suite F-100
Kirkland, WA 98034
(206) 820-0547
CT,NT,PM

Port Townsend

Jonathan Collin, M.D. **(DIPL)**
911 Tyler Street
Port Townsend, WA 98368
(206) 385-4555
CT,NT,PM

Seattle

Thomas E. Woodson, M.D. **(P)**
807 Medical Dental Bldg.
509 Olive Way
Seattle, WA 98101
(206) 682-4421
A,BA,DD,GER,NT,PM

Yakima

Murray L. Black, D.O. **(P)**
609 S. 48th Avenue
Yakima, WA 98908
(509) 966-1780
A,CT,FP,GP,OSM

WEST VIRGINIA

Beckley

Prudencio Corro, M.D. **(D/C)**
Box 630
Route 4
Beckley, WV 25801
(304) 252-0775
A,CT,RHI

Michael M. Kostenko, D.O. **(P)**
200 George Street, Ste 1
Beckley, WV 25801
(304) 253-2101
A,AC,CT,FP,OSM,PM

Charleston

Steve M. Zekan, M.D. **(P)**
1208 Kanawha Blvd., East
Charleston, WV 25301-2915
(304) 925-0579
CT,NT,PM,S

Follansbee

Albert Molisky, D.O. **(P)**
748 Main Street
Follansbee, WV 26037
(304) 527-1626
CT,FP,HYP,OSM

Iaeger

Ebb K. Whitley Jr., M.D. **(D/C)**
Box 540
Route 52
Iaeger, WV 24844
(304) 938-5357
A,CD,DIA,DD,GP,PM

Milwaukee

William J. Faber, D.O. **(P)**
6529 W. Fond du Lac Ave.
Milwaukee, WI 53218
(414) 464-7680
AC,CT,DD,NT,OSM,PM

Robert R. Stocker, D.O. **(DIPL)**
2525 N. Mayfair Road
Milwaukee, WI 53226
(414) 258-6282
BA,CT,GP

Necedah

Philip F. Mussari, M.D. **(P)**
P. O. Box 409
235 Main Street
Necedah, WI 54646
(608) 565-7401
BA,CT,GP

Oconomowoc

Robert R. Stocker, D.O. **(DIPL)**
1005 N. Lake Road
Oconomowoc, WI 53066
(414) 567-6933
BA,CT,GP

Williams Bay

Rathna Alwa, M.D. **(D/C)**
Box 1290
93 W. Geneva Street
Williams Bay, WI 53191
(414) 245-5566
AC,AR,BA,CT,HYP,IM

American College of Advancement in Medicine (ACAM) Physicians—International

AUSTRALIA

Gosford, N.S.W.

Heather M. Bassett, M.D. **(D/C)**
91 Donnison Street
Gosford, N.S.W. 2250
(043) 24 7388
CD,DD,GYN,NT,OSM,PMR

Labrador, Q'ld

Patrick Glen McCabe, M.D. **(P)**
Shoreacres, Whiting St.
Labrador, Q'ld 4215
(075) 326-427
CT,NT,PM

BELGIUM

De Panne

Andre Mistiaen, M.D. **(P)**
8 Dynastie Laan
8470 De Panne
32-58-41-48-48
AC,AU,DD,GER,NT,PM

BRAZIL

Manaus, Amazonas

F.M. de Souza Filho, M.D. **(P)**
Rua Natal 204 Adrianopolis
Manaus, Amazonas
92-2367670
CT

Osorio-RS

Jose Valdi de Souza, M.D. **(P)**
St. Mal Floriano 1012
s/Iron 1 to 9
Osorio-RS 95520
(051) 663-1269
CD,CT,DD,GP,GER,PM

Pelotas-RS

Antonio C. Fernandes, M.D. **(P)**
Rua Santa Tecla 470A
Pelotas, RS 96010
0532-224699
CD,CT,GER,GP,IM,PM

Porto Alegre

Moyses Hodara, M.D. **(P)**
Rua Vigario Jose Inacio
368, Sala 102
Porto Alegre-RS
(0512) 24-3557
CS,CT,DD,FP,GP,RHU

Carlos J.P. de Sa, M.D. **(P)**
Marcilio Dias - 1056
Porto Alegre-RS 90000
(0512) 33-48-32
CD,CT,DIA,HGL,S

Rio de Janeiro

Helion Povoa Filho, M.D. **(P)**
Rua Conde de Iraja 513
Botafogo
Rio de Janeiro, RJ 22271
(021) 2665491
CT,MM,Pathology

Walter J. dos Santos, M.D. **(P)**
Rua Visconde de Piraja
156, Sala 601-604
Rio de Janeiro, CEP 22410
55-21-267-3348
A,BA,CD,CT,DD,PM

Sao Paulo

Guilherme P. Deucher, M.D. **(P)**
Rua Borges Lagoa 1231
20 Andar
Sao Paulo, CEP 04038
57 11 157
CT,PM,S

Tuffik Mattar, M.D. **(P)**
Rua 7 de Abril 282
CJ 113
Sao Paulo 01044
255-5682 or 255-5992
CD,CT,DD,GER,IM,PM

Roberto E. Tullii, M.D. **(P)**
Al Gabriel Monteiro da Silva
1719
Sao Paulo
85-29692 or 88-18780
CT,Vascular Surgery

CANADA

Blythe

Richard W. Street, M.D. **(P)**
Box 100
Gypsy Lane
Blythe, ON N0M 1H0
(519) 523-4433
CP,NT,PM

Sarnia

Nazer Vellani, M.D. **(P)**
241 Wellington St.
Sarnia, ON N7T 1G9
(519) 344-6171
CT,NT,PM

Smiths Falls

Clare Minielly, M.D. **(D/C)**
33 Williams Street E.
Smiths Falls, ON K7A 1C3
(613) 283-7703
AN,CT,GP,NT

Willowdale

Paul Cutler, M.D. **(DIPL)**
4841 Yonge St., Ste B-4
Willowdale, ON M2N 5X2
(416) 733-3151
A,CT,NT

DENMARK

Aarhus

Kurt Christensen, M.D. **(P)**
Scandinavian Chelation Clinic
Fredenstorv 8-1
8000 Aarhus C
6-126141
AC,CT,GP,NT

Bruce P. Kyle, M.D. **(P)**
Scandinavian Chelation Clinic
Fredenstorv 8-1
8000 Aarhus C
6-126141
AC,AU,CT,IM,NT,PM

Skodsborg

Bo Mogelvang, M.D.
Pain Clinic
Strandvejen 134
2942 Skodsborg
02-80-79-79
CT

Vedbaek

Claus Hancke, M.D. **(P)**
Troeroedvej 71
DK-2950 Vedbaek
2-76-00-71
CT,FP,GP,NT,OSM,PM

Vejle

Knut T. Flytlie, M.D. **(P)**
Daemningen 70
7100 Vejle
05-822020
A,AC,AU,GP,OSM,PM

DOMINICAN REPUBLIC

Santo Domingo

Antonio Pannocchia, M.D. **(P)**
Ave. 27 de Febrero, Ste 201
Santo Domingo 6
565-3259
CT,NT,PM

ENGLAND

Pagham, West Sussex

Phillip Lebon, M.D. **(P)**
The Chelation Clinic
3 The Glade
Pagham
West Sussex P021 4SD
01-935-7368
CT,S

FRANCE

Rueil Malmaison

Bruno Crussol, M.D. **(D/C)**
2 Avenue Talma
92500 Rueil Malmaison
33-1-42-25-45-39
CT,NT,PM,S

GERMANY, WEST

Bad Fussing

Karl Heinz Caspers, M.D. **(P)**
Beethovenstrasse 1
D 8397 Bad Fussing
08531-21001 or 08531-21004
NT,PM

Rottach-Egern

Claus Martin, M.D. **(P)**
P. O. Box 244
8183 Rottach-Egern
8022-6415
CT,DD,GER

Werne

Fens-Ruediger Collatz, M.D. **(P)**
Fuerstenhofklinik
Fuerstenhof 2
D 4712 Werne
02389-3883
AC,CT,DD,GER,HO,PM

INDONESIA

Bandung

Benjamin Widjajakusuma, M.D.
(D/C)
Pasirkaliki 115
Bandung 40172
(022) 615277
CD,DIA,GER,IM,NT,PUD

Jakarta

Maimunah Affandi, M.D. **(DIPL)**
Jalan Gandaria 8, Ste 13
Kebayoran-Baru
Jakarta-Selatan
(021) 716927
CD,CT,DD,PD

Adjit Singh Gill, M.D. **(P)**
Jalan Tanah Abang V, #27A
Jakarta
(021) 357359
CD,CT,PM

Yahya Kisyanto, M.D. **(D/C)**
Cipto Hospital
71 Diponegoro
Jakarta, Indonesia
(021) 334636
CD,CT,DIA,GER,IM,PMR

MEXICO

Chihuahua

Humberto Berlanga Reyes, M.D.
(DIPL)
Antonio de Montes 2118
Col. San Felipe
Chihuahua, Chih. 31240
(95) 141-3-92-71
(95) 141-3-92-75
CT,GER,GP,PM

Ciudad Juarez

Humberto Berlanga Reyes, M.D.
(DIPL)
Insurgentes 2516
Ciudad Juarez, Chih. 32330
13-80-23
CT,GP,GER,PM

Rosa Elia Quintana, M.D. **(DIPL)**
Insurgentes 2516
Ciudad Juarez, Chih. 32330
13-80-23
CT,GP,GER,PM

Ensenada

David Mora Cuevas, M.D. **(P)**
Ave. Delante, #339
Ensenada, B.C.
(706) 676-2750
A,CT,DD,FP,NT,PM

Guadalajara-Jalisco

Eleazar A. Carrasco, M.D. **(P)**
Chapultepec Norte 140-203
Guadalajara-Jalisco 44600
25-16-55
A,CT,GP,GYN,OBS,S

Mexico City

Joel Torres Uscanga, M.D. **(P)**
Insurgentes SUR 513
Mexico City-11-D.F. 06170
5-64-33-89
A,CT,GP,S

N. Laredo, Tamps

Ruben Berlanga, M.D. **(P)**
Guerrero, #3435, NVO
Esq. Paseo Colon
N. Laredo, Tamps
(011) 52-871-40930
AU,CT,GER,P,PM

Tijuana

Rodrigo Rodriguez, M.D. **(P)**
Azucenas 15
Frac. del Prado
Tijuana, B.C.
(706) 681-3171
CD,CT,DD,GER,MM,PM

Torreon, Coahuila

Carlos Lopez Moreno, M.D. **(P)**
Tulipanes 475
Col. Torreon, Jardin
Torreon, Coahuila 27200
76-363
CT,NT,PM

NETHERLANDS

Leende

P. J. van der Schaar, M.D. **(DIPL)**
Renheide 2
Leende 5595XJ
31 4959-2232
CD,CT,DD,OME,S

Maastricht

Rob van Zandvoort, M.D. **(DIPL)**
Burg. Cortenstraat 26
6226 GV Maastricht
(043) 623474
CT,GP,NT,PM

Rotterdam

Robert T.H.K. Trossel, M.D.
(DIPL)
Zoutmanstraat 4
3012 EV Rotterdam
10-412-63-62
AR,CD,CT,DD,GP,GER

Utrecht

P.J.C. Riethoven, M.D. **(P)**
Ramstraat 27-A
3581 HD Utrecht 030-518951
GP

NEW ZEALAND

Auckland

Maurice B. Archer, D.O. **(P)**
P. O. Box 2981
Auckland 1
32-847
CT,NT,PM

Masterton

T.J. Baily Gibson, M.D. **(DIPL)**
P. O. Box 274
Masterton
(059) 81-250
A,CT,FP,OBS,OME

Mt. Maunganui

Michael E. Godfrey, M.D. **(DIPL)**
4 Dee Street
Mt. Maunganui
54-057 Tauranga
CT,FP,GP,MM,PM,OBS

Oxford, No. Canterbury

Ted Walford, M.D. **(P)**
122 Main Street
Oxford, No. Canterbury
0502-24488
CT,NT,PM

PHILIPPINES

Manila

Benjamin P. Aquino, M.D. **(P)**
Room 406, Singson Bldg.
P. Moraga, Binondo
Manila
47-41-05
AC,AU,CD,CT,IM,R

Rosa M. Ami Belli, M.D. **(P)**
PDC Bldg., Ste 303-501
1440 Taft Avenue
Manila
50-03-23
CT,HGL,NT,P

Leonides Lerma, M.D. **(P)**
#301, Pearl Garden
1700 M. Adriatico Malate
Manila
57-59-11
A,AC,AU,GER,P

Corazon Macawili-Yu, M.D. **(P)**
PDC Bldg., Ste 303-501
1440 Taft Avenue
Manila
50-03-23
CT,FP,GP,GYN,PD,PM

Remedios L. Reynoso, M.D. **(P)**
PDC Bldg., Ste 303-501
1440 Taft Avenue
Manila
50-03-23
CT,NT,PM

Quezon City

Efren V. de los Santos, M.D. **(P)**
201 E. Rodriguez Sr. Blvd.
Quezon City 3008
78-70-11 or 77-31-83
Surgery

SWITZERLAND

Montreux

Claude Rossell, M.D., Ph.D. **(P)**
Clinique Bon Port
1820 Montreux
21-6351-01
CT,NT,PM

Netstal (Glarus)

Walter Blumer, M.D. **(P)**
8754 Netstal
(Glarus bei Zurich)
058-61-28-46
CT
(Honorary Life Member)

TAIWAN (R.O.C.)

Taipei

Paul Lin, M.D. **(P)**
5, Lane 85 Sung Chiang Rd.
Taipei
(02) 507-2222 (Taipei)
Ext. 1003
CT

THAILAND

Bangkok

Ann Bhuket, M.D. **(P)**
48/6 Suanlamtong 2
Prakanong, Pratakorn Rd.
Bangkok 11
31-44-182
A,AC,CT,IM,PD

About the Author

Dr. Morton Walker works full time as a professional free-lance medical journalist and author. To date, his publications include over 1,300 magazine articles and clinical journal papers and 43 books. His books are published by Simon & Schuster, E.P. Dutton, The Putnam Publishing Group, M. Evans & Co., Prentice-Hall, Macmillan Publishing, Keats Publishing, Contemporary Books, Arco Publishing, Avery Publishing Group Inc., and others. He is the author of such bestsellers as *Sexual Nutrition*, *The Yeast Syndrome*, and *Chelation Therapy*.

In 1976 Dr. Walker won the Jesse H. Neal Editorial Achievement Award for the best ongoing series of articles published in an American magazine in the previous year. He has received eighteen additional writing awards in special medical fields. In 1977 he was presented with the Jesse H. Neal Editorial Achievement Award from the American Business Press Inc. for the best special issue of a magazine published in the United States in the previous year. Then in 1979 he won the Humanitarian Award from the American Academy of Medical Preventics, and in 1981 he later won the Orthomolecular Award from the Institute of Preventive Medicine.

After receiving ten awards for research and writing in the field of podiatry from the American Podiatry Association, including that profession's highest award (the 1962 William J. Stickel Gold Medal), Dr. Walker left almost seventeen years of successful practice as a doctor of podiatric medicine (D.P.M.) to pursue his true interest, medical journalism. He has been a professional medical writer since 1969. He also lectures around the country and has appeared on nearly 900 radio, television, and press interviews including *The Merv Griffin Show, The Joe Franklin Show, Kup's Show, AM Chicago, People Are Talking, Midday, Mid-Morning LA, Good Day LA, AM San Francisco, AM Weekend San Francisco,* and many more throughout Canada and the United States. His special writing and discussion topics are holistic health, orthomolecular medicine, and alternative methods of healing.

Dr. Walker actively participates on committees of the American Society of Journalists and Authors Inc., the premier organization of professional writers; he has been a member since 1974. He lives with his wife Joan in Stamford, Connecticut, and has three grown sons and five grandchildren.

The Chelation Way: The Complete Book of Chelation Therapy is the fourth book Dr. Walker has authored on this vital subject. His three previous texts, *The Healing Powers of Chelation Therapy, Chelation Therapy,* and *The Chelation Answer* have been cited by holistic health authorities as having already saved possibly a quarter of a million Americans and Canadians from going under the surgeon's knife for open heart surgery, carotid artery cleaning, and limb amputation, and from numerous fatal illnesses. Now, with the addition of *The Chelation Way: The Complete Book of Chelation Therapy,* many more people will learn how they can benefit from chelation therapy.

Index

Hardening of arteries, 30–31, 39,
   104
   arteriolar sclerosis, 30
   atherosclerosis, 30
   hypertensive arteriosclerosis,
   30
   Mönckeberg's medial
   arteriosclerosis, 30
Halstead, Dr. Bruce W., 29–30, 76,
   81, 97, 101, 157–158, 231
Harris, Dr. Robert, 125–127
Haskell, Dr. Robert, 8, 10, 12
HDL, 63
*Healing Powers of Chelation Therapy,
   The,* 129
Health Horizons Exposition, 34
Heart disease, 114, 128
Hemoglobin, 23, 102
Henck, Jack, 99
Herbs, 154, 217–245
Hexopal Forte, 225
High-density lipoprotein (HDL),
   63
Hills, Dr. Christopher, 237–238
Hirsh, Cheryl, 69–70
Histidine. *See* Amino acid.
Hohnbaum, Dr. Roland C.,
   162–165
Holistic medicine, 71, 156–158,
   239–240
Hollingsworth, Brunson, 187–190
Homeostasis, cellular, 156–158
Honeybee pollen, 169, 170,
   243–244
Hormone DHEA, 42
Horrobin, Dr. David, 240
Hume, Dr. R., 176
Hyperbaric oxygen, 20, 34
Hypercalcemia, 118
Hypertension, 59, 87
Hypertensive arteriosclerosis, 30
Hypocalcemia, 107

Hypoglycemia, 108, 120, 153
Hypotension, 108

Impotence, 49–50, 53, 130
Inderal, 20, 107, 130, 217
Indigestion, 212
Infarction. *See* Myocardial
   infarction.
Ingler Company, 183
Intravenous (IV) fluids. *See*
   Chelation therapy.
Investigational new drug (IND),
   127
Iodide. *See* Iodine.
Iodine (iodide), 181
Iordanidis, C., 169
Iridology, 119, 120
Iron, 168, 181. *See also* Poisons,
   metallic.
Ishikawa, Professor Masayuki,
   221–222
Isordil, 188

Johnson, Noel, 167–170, 244
Johnson, William D., 135
Journal of Advancement in Medicine,
   80
*Journal of American Medical
   Association* (JAMA), 95
*Journal of Applied Nutrition in
   Clinical Practice,* 233
Journal of Holistic Medicine, 77, 79,
   82, 137
*Journal of the International Academy
   of Preventive Medicine,* 82
*Journal of Osteopathic Physicians and
   Surgeons of California,* 83

Kanary, Elmer R., 123
Kenyon, Dr. Keith, 211–212,
   213–214
Key Company, 183
Kidney disease. *See* Nephrology.